M000118055

THYROID GUIDE TO HAIR LOSS:
A Comprehensive Guide to Hair Loss for Thyroid Patients

By

Mary J. Shomon

With Cynthia Austin

http://www.thyroid-info.com/hair

IMPORTANT NOTE

This guide does not provide medical advice, diagnosis or treatment. The contents of this guide, such as text, graphics, images, and other material contained in the guide ("Content") are for informational purposes only. The Content is not intended to be a substitute for professional medical advice, diagnosis, or treatment. Always seek the advice of your physician or other qualified health provider with any questions you may have regarding a medical condition. Never disregard professional medical advice or delay in seeking it because of something you have read in this guide!

This guide does not recommend or endorse any specific tests, physicians, products, procedures, opinions, or other information that may be mentioned. Reliance on any information provided by this guide is solely at your own risk.

If you think you may have a medical emergency, call your doctor or 911 immediately.

Links to Web sites other than those owned by Mary Shomon are offered as a service to readers. Mary Shomon was not involved in their production and is not responsible for their content.

> **Many thanks to Cynthia Austin for her tremendous research and writing effort, which was integral to the development of this ebook.**

THYROID GUIDE TO HAIR LOSS

TABLE OF CONTENTS

SECTION 3: HAIR LOSS TREATMENTS

APPENDICES

A NOTE FROM MARY SHOMON

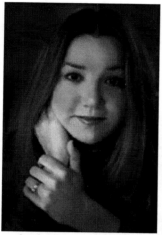

Your hair loss is making you miserable. I know that, because you've bought this Guide.

And truly, I know exactly how your feel.

I have always had a full head of hair – at least until my thyroid started acting up. Then, it seemed as if I could stuff pillows with the hair that came out during each shower. I went through bottles of Drano, unclogging my hair-filled drains. My hairbrushes looked like Chia-pets after each brushing!

To be honest, I dreaded just running my hands through my hair, because it seemed like each time I did so, 50 more hairs would fall out!

I was pretty sure I'd end up bald.

And the real moment of truth? When my usually thick ponytail became so thin that it was the thickness of a pencil! I remember my mother – and mothers always know, don't they! – looking at me and saying, "Mary, something's *really* wrong with your hair. It's half gone!"

I knew I had to do something.

So my regular doctor, perplexed and frustrated for me, sent me off for a consultation to a self-proclaimed "specialist" on thyroid disease, who told me that I was losing hair because I was "stressed out."

Darn right I was stressed out. I was stressed out because I was losing my hair!

But I knew the hair loss had started with my thyroid condition, and worsened when I was taking the drug Synthroid. Dr. "Expert" said that Synthroid had nothing to do with the hair loss.
I sat in the car and cried for an hour after that utterly useless appointment.

But the appointment wasn't totally useless. Because I was so frustrated and angry, I became motivated.

Motivated to study everything I could about thyroid disease and hair loss.

So I read dozens of pages on Synthroid and its side effects. I talked to experts. I researched alternative techniques.

And I found out what was likely worsening my hair loss.

And I took action.

And my hair loss stopped.

Then my hair started to fill back in.

And now, I have hair again.

In fact, here's a photo of my hair not too long ago. (Nothing fake, no hair extensions, just my own hair! – There is a bit of hair color on it though!)

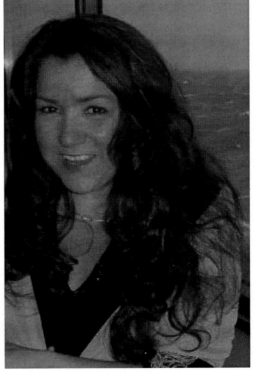

I can't promise that you'll have the same results, because hair loss has a variety of triggers, and we don't all respond the same to various treatments.

THYROID GUIDE TO HAIR LOSS

But I can promise you that after you read this guide, you'll understand hair loss, especially as it happens in thyroid patients. And you'll have an entire list of approaches to discuss with your practitioner, and try, to help deal with your hair loss.

No snake oil. No magic potions. No revolutionary techniques. Just facts from the world of conventional, holistic, and integrative medicine.

* * *

Before I continue, I'd like to explain my own background. I'm not a doctor or health professional. I have a degree in International Studies from Georgetown University. I never expected to be writing about health and thyroid disease, but back in 1995, at the age of 33, I was diagnosed with Hashimoto's disease, the autoimmune condition that causes hypothyroidism. The diagnosis was a turning point in my life and in my career, as I first launched an intensive effort to return to good health myself.

Later, I expanded my own research and information-gathering effort into a mission to share this knowledge, and a role as a patient advocate. In 1997, I started a popular, patient-oriented Web site on thyroid disease, http://www.thyroid-info.com, and became the Guide to Thyroid Disease for About.com http://thyroid.about.com, (a division of the *New York Times*.) These are sites I still run today, more than a decade after I started them.

In 1998, I launched the only independent print and email newsletters on thyroid health from a conventional and alternative perspective, called *Sticking Out Our Necks* (http://www.thyroid-info.com/subscribe.htm). I've also written a number of books and magazine articles to help people overcome health challenges. (See page the last section for a complete list of all my books.)

These days, I get hundreds of emails and letters each week from readers all over the world, sharing their stories and looking for solutions to their own thyroid and hormonal health challenges.

THYROID GUIDE TO HAIR LOSS

Because so many people have written in desperation, looking for help with hair loss problems, it seemed critical to write this ebook for the millions of you who, like me, deal with hair loss related to thyroid disease and hormones.

Many of you don't even know you have a thyroid problem yet, and for you, I hope this book can provide a roadmap that will help you move quickly through the process of recognizing your symptoms, getting diagnosed, and receiving proper treatment.

Finding and properly treating thyroid disease is of course not a complete solution for hair loss for everyone. But it is a solution for some of you, and the health and wellness benefits of getting an undiagnosed thyroid condition properly identified and treated are immeasurable.

There are also many people who, like me, have already been diagnosed and treated for a thyroid condition. But you may not realize that if your thyroid treatment is not the optimized and carefully monitored, your hair may pay the price.

And among thyroid patients, when hair loss continues, you need information.

There's a dizzying array of options – from prescription drugs, to lasers, to herbs, supplements, and more. But in this Guide, you'll learn about what works for thyroid patients, and what doesn't, so you can map out an effective plan!

I wish you all the best, and hope that this Guide is a start of your return to better health – and more hair!!

Live well,

Mary

**A hair in the head
is worth
two in the brush.**

~ Oliver Herford

SECTION 1
OVERVIEW

INTRODUCTION

Hair in the shower drain, your brush, or on your pillow in the morning does not necessarily signal a hair loss problem. The average person loses about 100 hairs a day (about enough to fully cover a shower drain). As we age, hair does thin and follicles do stop producing hair. It's a normal part of the aging process. It's almost guaranteed that as you get older, you will not have the same amount or thickness of hair that you had earlier in life.

But when significant hair loss or thinning occurs, let's face it: hair loss is traumatic.

You're reading this guide because you--or someone you care about--are struggling with hair loss. There's no question that hair loss can be frightening– and it's a problem made even worse by the vast array of theories, expensive products, and supplements of questionable value that are being touted as the latest, greatest cure for hair loss.

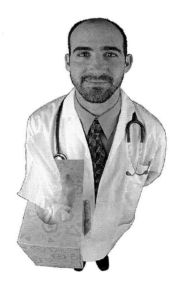

Whether you're a man or a woman, you can experience thinning hair or hair loss. And there are a number of reasons for hair that is thinning or falling out. These reasons are explored in this guide, along with a look at some of the solutions available to help.

Special attention is given to thyroid disease, a common yet frequently ignored health condition that affects an estimated 59 million Americans. Why is thyroid disease a special focus of this hair loss guide? Because hair loss is a common symptom and side effect of thyroid disease, yet many patients – and their doctors – do not recognize hair-related thyroid symptoms as connected to thyroid disease.

Many people suffering unexplained hair loss might in fact have *undiagnosed* thyroid conditions. Diagnosing and treating the thyroid condition may resolve the hair problems.

Find the thyroid problem, and treat it, and hair loss problem solved.

(And keep in mind, experts think that **the majority of thyroid sufferers – perhaps as many as 45 million Americans -- have *not* been diagnosed yet.**)

Even among thyroid patients receiving treatment, hair loss is still a common concern. And so the guide addresses the full range of hair loss causes and treatments for those of you in this situation as well.

Ultimately, the *Thyroid Guide to Hair Loss* gives you the information you need to make intelligent choices about the frustrating challenge of hair loss.

HAIR THROUGH HISTORY

Although we generally focus on hair loss in our day and age, it has affected humankind throughout history. While facial hair has dropped in and out of fashion for thousands of years, scalp hair has almost always been considered a symbol of vigor, youth and health. Even the Bible mentions baldness! And just like today, there have always been remedies and ointments available for those with the resources to buy them.

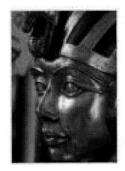

One of the oldest prescriptive medical documents known is a 110 page scroll known as the Ebers Papyrus that dates back to 1500 BC. Included in the scroll is a remedy for hair loss that recommends consuming a blend of iron, lead, honey and alabaster, all while reciting a prayer. Hippocrates, the Greek doctor who was born in 460 BC and became known as the "Father of Medicine," recommended a baldness treatment that involved applying pigeon droppings and opium to the scalp.

And thousands of years later, they're *still* trying to sell us some pretty wild cures for hair loss! But, unlike our hair-challenged ancestors, ongoing research has unlocked some of the secrets behind hair loss and given us some viable treatment options.

When you're going through any hair loss, it can be devastating. Hair is a key part of our physical appearance, and it can also serve as expression of our attractiveness, virility, and general health. What is biologically there for warmth and scalp protection is now fundamental to self-esteem and the image we project to other people. You need only turn on the television or pick up a magazine to find celebrities, models, or sports figures – usually with a full head of healthy hair. Attractive hair is associated with youth, intelligence, attractiveness and sex appeal in our society, while baldness is considered a topic to laugh about.

Both men and women have some loss of hair and thinning with age. And while it may seem that men are most affected, the American Academy of Dermatology notes that about half of the women in the United States experience some type of hair loss by age 50.

Dr. Valerie Callender, a clinical assistant professor at Howard University College of Medicine says:

> By age 40, visible symptoms of female pattern hair loss are present in 40 percent of women. Since society has placed a great deal of social and cultural importance on hair and hairstyles, hair loss in women can be devastating.

Studies actually suggest that the psychological and social effects of hair loss are greater in women than in men. For women, hair loss can even lead to social withdrawal, anxiety and a higher prevalence of personality disorders. All this is to say, for women, losing hair is especially

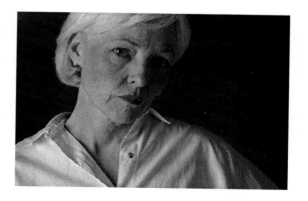

stressful!

That doesn't mean that men don't find losing their hair a frustrating and embarrassing experience as well. Some men begin to see evidence of male pattern balding in their early twenties, and men of all ages can experience a loss of self-confidence, depression and anxiety due to thinning hair or a receding hairline.

For both sexes, hair loss, whether permanent or temporary can be frightening and unwelcome. Although hair loss is not physically debilitating it can be emotional damaging at any point in life. Studies have shown that dealing with hair loss can, in some people, feel similar to dealing with a more serious, life-threatening disease.

FACTS ABOUT FOLLICLES

The hair follicles that serve throughout your lifetime are formed in the first trimester of pregnancy. Although no new follicles are formed after birth, the size, color and cyclical activity of the follicle all change throughout life. There are hair follicles all over the body but the greatest number reside on your scalp.

On average, there are 100,000 to 150,000 follicles in the scalp area with some variation in number owing to natural coloring – for example, individuals with natural blonde hair usually have about 140,000 hairs, brunettes 105,000 and redheads approximately 90,000 hairs.

At skin level, there is an opening to the hair follicle called a pore. The hair follicle itself is positioned at an angle in the scalp. A muscle is attached to the side of each follicle and when the muscle contracts, the hair stands up, resulting in a "goose bump." Within the follicle is a hair shaft and an oil gland called a sebaceous gland. The oil gland produces sebum that removes old cells, conditions the scalp and lessens water loss from skin tissues.

At the root of the hair shaft is a pouch-like structure called a follicle. Think of the shape of a temperature thermometer. Blood vessels in the bulb at the bottom nourish cells in the hair follicle. The follicle is composed of several cell layers that are some of the fastest growing cells in the human body.

The hair shaft grows out of the bulb at the bottom and extends beyond the skin surface where we can see it. Hair follicles are a rich, complicated environment.

They cycle throughout the lifetime, regenerating themselves based on unique molecular communications with sites and substances throughout the body.

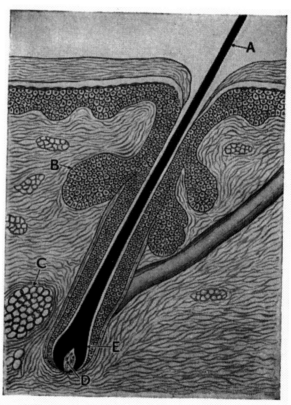

GREATLY ENLARGED ROOT OF A HUMAN HAIR
(A) Hair; (B) oil glands; (C) growing cells; (D) papilla (connective tissue which extends into and nourishes the roots of a hair); (E) hair follicle (the depression from which the hair grows).

HOW HAIR GROWS

Each hair follicle works on an asynchronous cycle, that is, a routine independent of the root follicle cells around it. There are three cycles of hair growth that affect individual hair follicles.

- At any time, about 90% of hair follicles are in the growth or *anagen* stage, which can last on average four to five years. Some experts divide the anagen period into two stages – early and late.

- In the *catagen* phase, cell growth and pigmentation stops and the hair begins to transition – the shaft stops growing and the outer sheath of the hair shaft shrinks and attaches to the root of shaft.

- In the *telogen* phase, hair growth ceases.

About 10% of hair follicles are in a transition or resting stage at any given time and this period can last several months. At the end of the resting phase, the hair shaft falls out and is replaced by a new hair. Thus, some hair loss is normal. Approximately 50 to 100 hairs may be shed on a usual day. The cycling of the hair follicle is genetically determined and most cases of hair loss are caused by disturbances in this phased cycling of the hair follicle. The factors that affect this "hair clock cycle" are not well understood.

Thinning occurs when either more hair falls out than is replaced by new hair, or individual hair shafts miniaturize, becoming smaller or thinner and allowing more scalp to show through. Instead of the larger, thicker terminal hair, the texture of hair may become soft and shorter in length. This type of usually colorless hair is called *vellus* hair.

Baldness occurs when hair falls out that is not replaced by new hair.

Hair grows about a half-inch a month or on average, about six inches a year, but this rate slows with age. Individuals who are able to grow their hair longer in length have a more extended growing, or anagen phase, than individuals whose hair stops growing at shorter lengths. Shorter hairs found on the body, such as eyebrows, eyelashes have a short anagen stage, which accounts for their shorter length.

Interestingly, studies note that hair and beard growth is greatest in the warmer parts of the year. For instance, facial and scalp hair growth peaks in September with a corresponding slowdown in growth in colder months such as December or January.

> **People get real comfortable with their features. Nobody gets comfortable with their hair. Hair trauma. It's the universal thing.**
> ~ Jamie Lee Curtis

Hair growth occurs in the base of the follicle, where the cells divide rapidly. The hair shaft itself is composed of a protein called keratin, which is organized in three layers, the cuticle, cortex and medulla. Keratin is the same substance that forms finger and toenails, hair, animal horns and hooves.

The outer layer of the hair shaft, the cuticle, looks like overlapping or stacked scales when viewed closely and the cuticle is the layer that may be affected by hair care products. Because the cells that form it overlap, the cuticle reflects light and gives hair shine or gloss as it protects the hair shaft. If the outer cuticle of the hair shaft becomes damaged, the overlapping scales lift up, exposing the dull cortex layer beneath and allowing moisture to escape. When damaged, the scales will also catch on each other, causing hair to tangle easily.

Keratin is colorless, so specialized cells called melanocytes produce the pigment in granules, located in the hair shaft, and give hair its color. The more melanin and the more granules, the darker the hair color will be. When the melanocytes cease producing melanin, the hair shaft will emerge gray and eventually white.

CAUSES OF HAIR LOSS

Hair loss is a complicated issue. There are different types of hair loss, and and no one thing causes all types of hair loss.

There are many myths about hair loss as well. Here are a few facts, for example, to counteract the popular myths:

- Hair loss is *not* the result of wearing hats, even tight hats.

- Brushing hair 100 strokes before bed won't help -- or hurt -- the abundance of your hair.

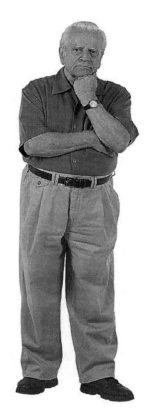

- Hair loss cannot be prevented or assisted with topical follicle cleansing preparations…follicles are located *under* the skin.

- Hanging upside down or standing on your head won't help hair loss.

- Cutting or shaving your head does not make your hair grow back faster or thicker.

Alopecia is the medical term for hair loss. There are several types of hair loss. For example, hair loss can be caused by an underlying or undiagnosed physical condition such as thyroid problem, lupus or diabetes. Hair loss can result from nutritional deficiencies. Hair loss can be the side effect of medications, such as therapies used to treat cancer. Hair loss is also common after childbirth, and during menopause.

While certain nutritional supplements may (or may not) be a factor in retaining hair, overuse of certain supplements can cause hair to fall out. Stress can also be a factor in hair loss, as we will discuss later.

Hair loss can also result from poisoning, such as with high blood levels of mercury in people who overconsume contaminated fish.

(Overconsumption of certain types of fish – especially shark, swordfish, king mackerel, or tilefish, for example -- can sometimes cause mercury toxicity and resulting hair loss.)

THYROID GUIDE TO HAIR LOSS

> **NOTE: If you experience rapid onset, sudden loss of hair, consult a physician.**

Let's take a look at different forms of hair loss and factors of their development.

ANDROGENETIC ALOPECIA

Hereditary hair loss, called androgenetic alopecia ("AGA"), is the most common form of hair loss, and it is not contagious. It is also known as male- or female-pattern hair loss. If your hair is starting to thin, you may blame your maternal grandfather, who is bald. However, the genetic tendency toward hair loss can be inherited from either line of your family, including your own mother or father.

Androgenetic alopecia affects both genders and all ethnicities. It can begin as early as the teen years – anytime after puberty -- or not until later in life. AGA may not become evident until a person reaches his or her fifties.

Although not completely understood, hormones and their behavior are considered to be a prime factor in hair loss. A 2004 study noted that hair phase cycling is affected by sex hormones (estrogen, progesterone), thyroid, adrenal, pituitary and pineal hormones. A specific category of hormones known as "androgens" are known to be involved in androgenetic alopecia.

Testosterone is a type of androgen hormone. The production of one type of testosterone, dihydrotestosterone ("DHT") -- is thought to be a fundamental factor in AGA. In this type of loss, hair follicles begin to produce an enzyme known as 5-alpha reductase. When testosterone that is already present in the hair follicle combines with 5-alpha reductase, it creates DHT. Receptors located in hair follicles react to DHT by interrupting the hair phase cycle and signaling a reduction in follicle size. This causes changes in hair texture, diameter and length.

You can see that even though each hair follicle may have adequate blood supply to nourish the follicle, the effect of androgen hormones -- or other as yet undiscovered factors -- can cause the follicle to miniaturize, and may eventually cause hair growth from that follicle to stop.

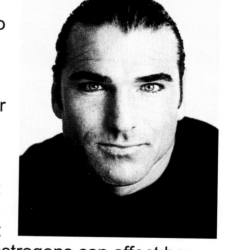

Though fewer studies address estrogen and the hair growth cycle, the involvement and metabolism of the estrogen group of hormones may prove as significant as that of androgens. Research has shown that estrogens can affect how the way follicles handle androgen hormones. With many key questions unanswered involving hair biology and estrogens, it is likely this will be a fruitful area of research in the future.

AGA is characterized by a shortening of the hair's growth cycle, a progressive shortening and thinning of individual hair shafts and may progress until no hair growth is evident. AGA is not associated with redness, itching or pain, nor is it technically considered a medical disorder.

Male pattern hair loss typically begin with a reduction in hair at the temples that proceeds back to the crown and appears as an "M" shape when viewed from above. Eventually, remaining hair may take the form of a ring or horseshoe that rims the head on the sides and back of the scalp. It is generally accepted that the earlier in life that male pattern hair loss is experienced, the more profound hair loss will be.

According to the American Medical Association, male pattern hair loss affects approximately 40 million men in the United States. While testosterones (and thus eventually DHT) are the androgens that increase the size of hair follicles in the beard and underarm area in men during puberty, they are also responsible for the decrease in follicle size of scalp hair later in life.

Female pattern hair loss may be significant, but is often easier to hide than the more commonly seen male pattern balding. In women, the hairline is not usually affected, but hair is lost in a more diffuse pattern. Hair is lost or thinned on the crown of the head in a "Christmas tree" pattern when viewed from above. Hair becomes finer and hairs are smaller or miniaturized, and the scalp becomes easier to see.

Some women experience AGA as early as their twenties, but it's much more common around menopause, after which as many as 37% of women experience hair loss and thinning.

Some women are sensitive to androgens. Women with androgen sensitivity disorders – such as Polycystic Ovarian Syndrome (POS) -- may also experience irregular menstrual periods or hirsutism (excessive hair growth on their upper lip and face). Blood tests can

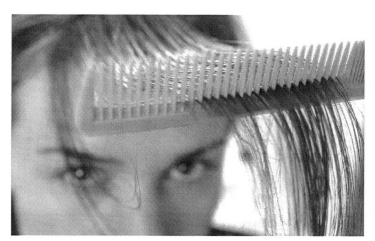

determine androgen sensitivity. Hair loss in women sensitive to androgens may also be the first sign of diabetes.

Genetics, hormones and aging combine to form a potent, but common trio in androgenetic alopecia.

There also seems to be some increased risk of AGA in thyroid patients. The relationship between AGA and the thyroid is discussed in depth later in this guide.

ALOPECIA AREATA

Alopecia Areata ("AA") is a complicated autoimmune disorder that can cause mild to severe hair loss on the scalp and body, sometimes for months and years. The disorder can be traced back to ancient times, and was named "alopecia areata" around 1760 to refer to "baldness in spots." AA affects people of all ages and both genders, though it appears more commonly in children. The National Alopecia Areata Foundation estimates that AA will affect approximately 4.5 million people in the United States during their lifetimes.

The term "autoimmune" disorder refers to a condition where the immune system attacks the body's own tissues, cells, organs, and glands. Experts don't really know why we develop autoimmune diseases, but we do know that for some reason, the body stops being able to tell the difference between our own body (and our cells, tissues, etc.), compared to foreign substances such as viruses or bacteria. With an autoimmune disorder, the body sends antibodies – usually produced to fight the viruses or bacteria – to instead attack our own tissues or organs. Gradually, the antibodies inflame, and in some cases, even destroy their target.

With AA, hair follicles are mistakenly attacked by the body's own white blood cells. This assault on the hair follicles causes hair cells to shrink ("miniaturize," in medical speak) and they slow down and eventually stop producing hair. While white blood cells attack hair follicles, they do not attack stem cells that create new hair cells, so regrowth of hair *is* possible.

While AA usually manifests as round or patchy hair loss on the scalp, less commonly, it leads to a total loss of hair on the scalp ("alopecia totalis") or the body ("alopecia universalis").

AA is not contagious, and doesn't typically have any physical symptoms beyond hair loss. Many germs, bacteria and viruses are screened out by eyelashes, eyebrows, nose and ear hair, so the loss of facial hair can leave a sufferer more vulnerable to infection.

AA can be an emotionally devastating condition for people of any age. As many as three-fourths of all alopecia patients may suffer from some sort of anxiety, depression, or mental health issue as a result of their AA.

Adding to the frustration of the disorder, the course of AA is unpredictable. Hair may regrow and then fall out again months or years later. Regrown hair may be white, but usually returns to normal texture and pigmentation over time.

There is currently no cure for AA, nor medications specifically approved to treat it. Using hair regrowth medications that are approved for pattern hair loss may be effective initially, but they do not treat the underlying cause of the hair loss, and thus episodes of AA-triggered hair loss are likely to recur. However, there are treatments and medications that are used to assist in the growth of hair, whether it is retained or not.

An important note: Hair lost to AA that is regrown under the influence of medications will be lost when treatment ceases.

Corticosteroids are sometimes used in the treatment of AA. Another drug that is used is minoxidil (also known by its brand name, Rogaine.) Other drugs and treatments used for AA include anthralin, sulfasalazine, cyclosporine, photochemotherapy ("PUVA")-and topical sensitizers.

On the alternative front, a small 2002 study found that treatment with topically applied onion juice assisted in regrowth of hair in AA patients. A 1998 study found that aromatherapy treatment with certain essential oils was successful for some AA sufferers.

As noted, because autoimmune disorders are not fully understood, it is not known specifically what causes AA. While genetics and hereditary are thought to be risk factors, so are life stressors such as emotional loss, or situations and conditions that stress the body, such as pregnancy or exposure to a virus, bacteria or environmental toxin.

AA is, however, hereditary in part. In identical twin studies— identical twins being individuals who share the same genes— 55% of twin sets experience AA. This suggests that while heredity is a factor, it does not entirely explain the development of AA. We do know that the earlier the onset of AA, the more likely that it will affect other family members at some point in their lives.

There is also a connection between AA and other autoimmune diseases. Having AA does not mean that an individual is going to develop another autoimmune disease. People with AA do, however, have a higher incidence of some disorders, such as allergies, asthma or thyroid problems.

And having a personal or family history of other autoimmune disorders -- such as Hashimoto's disease, Graves' disease, multiple sclerosis, systemic lupus erythematosus or rheumatoid arthritis, for example – also puts you at a higher risk for AA.

There is, as noted, a specific connection between thyroid disease and AA. Some researchers have found evidence of thyroid antibodies in AA patients, and these patients also tend to have a substantially higher risk of thyroid problems. The relationship between AA and the thyroid is discussed in depth later in this guide.

TELOGEN EFFLUVIUM

Telogen effluvium ("TE") is a relatively common type of hair loss characterized by increased shedding over the entire scalp. Hair loss is noticeable -- when combing, brushing and washing hair as well as on the pillow in the morning. It affects both genders and is not contagious.

"Acute" TE resolves within six months, whereas "chronic" TE is defined as generalized shedding that does not resolve within six months.

There are a number of causes of TE, including:

- Hormonal changes related to pregnancy -- During pregnancy, an increase in estrogen and progesterone can cause changes in hair texture and quantity. During the postpartum period women may notice they are shedding more hair than they did in previous months. This type of TE is normal and will gradually cease as the body resumes a non-pregnant physiological cycle.

- Sudden physiological changes (such as those brought about by crash dieting)

- Illness. The onset or an episode of an disease such as thyroid disease, lupus, diabetes, or rheumatoid arthritis can also be an underlying cause of TE.

- Toxin overexposure/poisoning. TE can be caused by poisoning or overexposure to substances such as selenium or arsenic.

- A physical stressor/shock, such as surgery, or an accident.

- Certain medications, for example oral contraceptives, beta-blockers, anticoagulants, medication for cystic acne, some anti-depressants, anti-seizure drugs, and levothyroxine (synthetic thyroid hormone replacement)

- Vaccinations have been reported to cause acute TE in some people

In addition to physical stress, acute or chronic emotional or psychological stress can be a primary cause of TE. A 2003 study found that hormones released when the body is under stress have a significant effect on the cycling of hair follicles, and on the hair shaft itself.

Stress hormones affect the hair follicle by causing hair to enter the catagen (transition) stage prematurely, bringing on the resting (telogen) stage of the follicle earlier than normal. Hair follicles shifted into a resting stage then thin and eventually fall out. TE does not generally cause bald patches, instead, you'll see significant overall thinning of scalp hair. Hair loss caused by TE can last an indeterminate amount of time, depending upon the underlying cause.

While TE usually resolves itself over time, in terms of treatment, minoxidil (Rogaine) is known to prolong the anagen (growing) stage of the hair cycle, but its effectiveness in offsetting the effects of stress hormones is unknown. It is clear that for individuals suffering from TE, comprehensive management of symptoms and underlying factors, such as nutritional deficiencies, should be considered. Hair-loss promoting medications should be evaluated. Non-pharmacological options such as counseling and mind-body approaches for stress and anxiety reduction may also be useful.

> **Stress related to dealing with another physical condition can worsen hair loss. So people who are already dealing with androgenetic alopecia or alopecia areata, and who experience significant emotional stress about it, can actually worsen their hair loss.**

ANAGEN EFFLUVIUM

Anagen effluvium ("AE") is hair loss usually caused by medications — chemotherapy drugs, for example -- and other drugs or poisons as discussed earlier. These substances damage the metabolic ability of hair follicles that are in the growing (anagen) stage of their production cycle. This type of hair loss is not contagious.

The use of minoxidil is often recommended with medication-induced AE. Minoxidil will not prevent hair loss, but it can shorten the period of hair loss and baldness that follows treatment by chemotherapy. When diagnostically appropriate, another technique to help reduce the amount of hair loss with cancer treatment is the use of a pressure cuff and cooling of the scalp during administration of the chemotherapy. Slowing the circulation of blood throughout the scalp reduces the amount of medication reaching susceptible hair follicles.

Again, this will not prevent hair loss, but may reduce the amount of hair lost.

Hair lost to AE will regrow as soon as the medications or poisons that are causing it are no longer circulating in the body. Hair follicles are not damaged by chemotherapy and will grow hair again, though hair may be a different color and texture than before treatment.

**Fair tresses man's imperial race
ensnare, and beauty draws us
with a single hair.**
~ Alexander Pope

LESS COMMON HAIR LOSS CONDITIONS

Cicatricial Alopecia

Primary cicatricial alopecia is an uncommon hair loss disorder caused by inflammation in the hair follicle's stem cells and oil glands. Another type of cicatricial alopecia is referred to as secondary cicatricial alopecia, and is caused when part of the scalp is destroyed by illness, tumor, radiation or injury. The term "cicatricial" means the hair loss is scarring. Damaged hair follicles are replaced by non-hair producing scar tissue. Hair lost to cicatricial alopecia is, therefore, permanently lost.

With primary cicatricial alopecia there are two predominant types of inflammatory cells that attack the hair follicle. These are known as *lymphocytes* and *neutrophils*. Treatment of the condition is based upon the type of active inflammatory cell. Neither type of cicatricial alopecia is contagious.

As noted, cicatricial alopecia is uncommon, but can affect both men and women, usually younger adults. One type of cicatricial alopecia, called frontal fibrosing alopecia, is more common in postmenopausal women, whereas central centrifugal alopecia affects primarily African American women.

Unlike other forms of hair loss, cicatricial alopecia can be painful, with itching, soreness, scaling, and redness of the scalp. Like AA, the course of cicatricial alopecia is unpredictable and may be lengthy. Cicatricial alopecia may appear and resolve only to reappear a year or two following.

Studies have shown that inflammatory cells that destroy stem cells and the sebaceous gland in the upper portion of the hair shaft destroy the follicle itself. Currently no cure exists for this frustrating disorder, but research moves forward in the development of diagnostic criteria that might allow the condition to be identified earlier, before follicle destruction occurs.

Since the progression of the condition causes permanent hair loss, it is important to seek qualified medical treatment from an experienced dermatologist quickly, in order to determine and begin a course of treatment. Treatment can include the use of anti-inflammatory medications, corticosteroids, antibiotics and other medications.

Tinea Capitis

Tinea capitis is a fungus, known more commonly as "ringworm." It is most often found in children 3 to 7 years of age, but can also be found in other age groups, with the risk dropping after puberty.

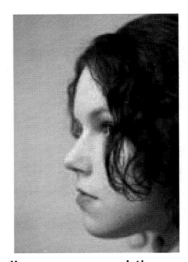

Tinea is contagious. Tinea capitis was once spread primarily by pets, especially cats, but the incidence of human-spread tinea is rising in North America and Europe. It can be spread between family members and friends sharing headgear, combs or brushes. In adults, hair shaving, braiding and certain hair oils may spread the transmission of the fungus.
Like most fungi, tinea capitis thrives in warm most spots such as the scalp. Increased risk factors include poor hygiene, prolonged wetness from sweating, and minor scalp injury.

Tinea capitis must be diagnosed and treated by a doctor. Tinea capitis must be diagnosed and treated by a doctor. The treatment is usually oral fungal medication and medicated shampoos. Left untreated, tinea capitis can lead to permanent hair loss via scarring of the scalp. Left untreated, tinea capitis can lead to permanent hair loss via scarring of the scalp.

Traction Alopecia

Traction alopecia is a type of hair loss caused by stress on the hair shaft. Traction alopecia is not contagious.

Traction alopecia is becoming increasingly common among young women due to the use of hair-weaving and hair extensions that require the existing hair shafts to carry the weight of additional synthetic or natural hair. Traction alopecia is also caused by tight braiding, cornrows, ponytails and any style or device that creates a continued pulling on the hair shaft. As noted, the hair loss is caused by pulling on the hair shaft, hair loss is not caused by compression, such as the wearing of hats or scarves.

If you are noticing thinning or balding spots on your scalp, make sure that your preferred hair style is not the culprit. Hair loss caused by traction alopecia is reversible once the cause of the tension is removed.

SECTION 2
THE THYROID CONNECTION

A MATTER OF BALANCE: THE THYROID AND YOUR HAIR

There's hope for hair loss in many people.

And it comes from your thyroid -- a small gland that is very powerful, but very often overlooked when it comes to women's hormonal complaints.

Your thyroid is a bowtie or butterfly-shaped gland located in your neck, below and behind the Adam's Apple area.

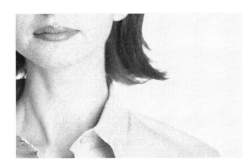

The thyroid is the master gland of energy and metabolism. The thyroid is also a key player in our complex and interconnected endocrine system, where it interacts with other endocrine glands such as the pancreas, adrenals, ovaries, and pituitary.

The thyroid releases hormones, and thyroid hormone rises and falls in concert with other endocrine hormones like insulin, cortisol, estrogen, and testosterone, among others.

Before you say, "But I don't think I have a thyroid problem," think again.

http://www.thyroid-info.com/hair

THYROID GUIDE TO HAIR LOSS

Thyroid disease is the most common autoimmune condition in America today. Thyroid problems are also common in many other countries, in particular, areas covered at one time by glaciers, where iodine is not present in the soil and in foods. In many of these countries, an enlarged thyroid, known as goiter, is seen is as many as one in five people, and is usually due to iodine deficiency.

Around the world, an estimated 8% of the population has goiter, most commonly women. In general, women are **seven times more likely than men to develop thyroid problems**. A woman, in fact, faces as much as a one in five chance of developing a thyroid problem during her lifetime.

The risk of thyroid disease increases with age, and by the age of 74, the prevalence of subclinical hypothyroidism in men, 16%, is nearly as high as the 21% rate seen in women.

Even the most conservative standards estimate that almost 27 million people have thyroid conditions in the U.S. And more than half of them are undiagnosed.

And this estimate may be just the tip of the iceberg...a vast underestimate actually.

Since 2002, experts in the endocrinology community have been calling for changes to the testing values that define "normal" thyroid function. While a minority of doctors already use the new standards for diagnosis and treatment, many practitioners have yet to adopt them.

http://www.thyroid-info.com/hair

THYROID GUIDE TO HAIR LOSS

When these changes are eventually followed across the board in laboratories and doctor's offices around the nation, approximately **59 million Americans will be considered to have thyroid disease.**

So, what this means is that, right now, according to the recommended standards, there are **as many as 40 million or more Americans with thyroid conditions of varying severity who don't know even they have a thyroid problem.**

Millions more have diagnosed and treated thyroid disease, but may still struggle with related symptoms and side effects.

However you look at it, there are millions of people who are experiencing hair loss and who are thyroid problems – but don't know it!

You may have in your mind what many consider the stereotypical thyroid patient...a middle aged, overweight woman. And if that's not you, you might assume you can't have a thyroid condition.

Or, you may think that only if you have an enlarged thyroid -- known as a goiter -- or bulging eyes could you have a thyroid problem. You may have even been told by a doctor, as one young mother was, "You can't possibly have a thyroid problem, because if you did, you wouldn't have been able to just have a baby!"

But being of normal weight, having a normal neck or eyes, or the fact that you were able to have a baby do not rule out a thyroid problem.

WHAT IS THE THYROID?

Your thyroid is a small bowtie or butterfly-shaped gland, located in your neck around the windpipe, behind and below your Adam's Apple area.

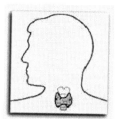

The thyroid, which is considered the master gland of metabolism, produces several hormones: triiodothyronine (T3) – the chief hormone at the cellular level -- and thyroxine (T4), which is converted to T3 before it reaches the cells. These hormones help oxygen get into your cells, and are critical to your body's ability to produce and use energy. **This role in delivering oxygen and energy makes your thyroid the master gland of metabolism.**

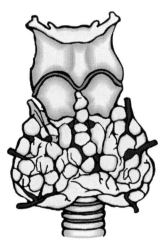

The Thyroid Gland

The thyroid has cells that are the only cells in the body capable of absorbing iodine. The thyroid takes in the iodine, obtained through food, iodized salt, or supplements, and combines that iodine with the amino acid tyrosine. The thyroid then converts the iodine/tyrosine combination into the hormones T3 and T4. The "3" and the "4" refer to the number of iodine molecules in each thyroid hormone molecule.

When it's in good condition, of all the hormones produced by your thyroid, 80% will be T4 and 20% T3. T3 is considered the biologically more active hormone -- the one that actually functions at the cellular level -- and is also considered several times stronger than T4.

Once released by the thyroid, the T3 and T4 travel through the bloodstream. The purpose is to help cells convert oxygen and calories into energy and serve as the basic fuel of your metabolism. As mentioned, the thyroid produces some T3. But the rest of the T3 needed by the body is actually formed from the mostly inactive T4 by a process sometimes referred to as "T4 to T3 conversion." This conversion of T4 to T3 can take place in some organs other than the thyroid, including the hypothalamus, a part of your brain.

As thyroid hormone circulates through your bloodstream, it attaches to and enters your cells via receptor sites on the membrane of the cells. Once inside the cell, thyroid hormone increases the cell's metabolic rate, including body temperature, and stimulates the cells to produce a number of different hormones, enzymes, neurotransmitters and muscle tissue. Thyroid hormone also helps your cells use oxygen and release carbon dioxide, which helps smooth metabolic function.

So how does the thyroid know how much thyroid hormone to produce? The release of hormones from the thyroid is part of a feedback process. The hypothalamus, a part of the brain, secretes Thyrotropin-Releasing Hormone (TRH). The release of TRH tells your pituitary gland to in turn produce Thyroid Stimulating Hormone (TSH).

I could announce one morning that the world was going to blow up in three hours and people would be calling in about my hair!
~ Katie Couric

http://www.thyroid-info.com/hair

This TSH, circulating in your bloodstream, is the messenger that tells your thyroid to make the thyroid hormones - the T4 and T3 – sending them into your bloodstream. When there is enough thyroid hormone circulating in your bloodstream, the pituitary makes *less* TSH, which is a signal to the thyroid that it can slow down hormone production. It's a smoothly functioning system -- *when it works properly*. When something interferes with the system and the feedback process doesn't work, thyroid problems can develop.

Thyroid Disease

There are actually two different autoimmune diseases that target the thyroid - Graves' disease, which causes an overactive thyroid (hyperthyroidism), and Hashimoto's thyroiditis, which causes an underactive thyroid (hypothyroidism).

In Graves' disease, autoantibodies bind to the thyroid gland, and cause the thyroid to overproduce thyroid hormone – the condition known as hyperthyroidism. Graves' disease is more common in women, and most frequently appears between the ages of 20-30. It's estimated that 3 million people have Graves' disease worldwide, with around 1.5 million in the United States. Usually, Graves' disease triggers hyperthyroidism, causing the gland to produce too much thyroid hormone. When hyperthyroid, your body goes into overdrive, gets sped up, causing an increased heart rate, increased blood pressure, and burning more calories more quickly.

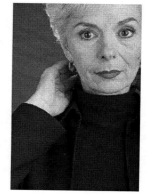

Hashimoto's thyroiditis can also be referred to as autoimmune thyroiditis, or chronic lymphocytic thyroiditis. In Hashimoto's, antibodies are reacting against proteins in the thyroid, causing gradual destruction of the gland itself, and its ability to produce the thyroid hormones the body needs. Eventually, most patients with Hashimoto's disease become hypothyroid, and the thyroid is underactive, and unable to produce enough hormone.

According to the American Autoimmune Related Diseases Association, as many as 25 percent of patients with Hashimoto's may also develop additional conditions, such as pernicious anemia, diabetes, adrenal insufficiency, or other autoimmune diseases.

Most people with autoimmune thyroid disease end up hypothyroid, the situation where the thyroid is either underactive, totally unable to function, or has been surgically removed. Hashimoto's thyroiditis usually slowly destroys the thyroid. Treatments for hyperthyroidism -- such as radioactive iodine (RAI) treatment, and surgical removal of the thyroid -- also usually result in hypothyroidism.

COULD YOU HAVE A THYROID PROBLEM? LET'S FIND OUT!

Risk factors for thyroid disease include the following:

- You have a personal or family history of thyroid problems
- You have a personal or family history of autoimmune disease (i.e., rheumatoid arthritis, psoriasis, vitiligo, multiple sclerosis, lupus, or other conditions)
- You are or were a smoker

- You have allergies or sensitivity to gluten, or diagnosed celiac disease

- You've been exposed to radiation, by living near or downwind from a nuclear plant, or through particular medical treatments (i.e., treatment for Hodgkins disease, nasal radium therapy, radiation to tonsils and neck area), or were near/downwind of the Chernobyl nuclear disaster in 1986

- You've been treated with lithium or amiodarone

- You have been taking supplemental iodine, kelp, bladderwrack, and/or bugleweed

- You live in an area (i.e., the Midwestern "Goiter Belt") where there is low iodine in the soil, and you have cut down on the iodized salt in your diet, leaving you iodine deficient

- You've been exposed to certain chemicals (i.e., perchlorate) via your water, food, or employment

- You've been excessively exposed to metals, such as mercury, and toxins such as environmental estrogens and pesticides

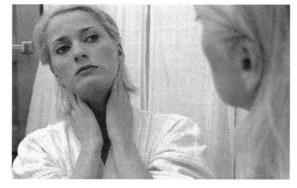

- You use fluoridated water and have dental fluoride treatments

- You are a heavy consumer of isoflavone-intensive soy products, especially soy powders or soy-based supplements

- You eat a substantial quantity of raw "goitrogenic" foods -- brussels sprouts, rutabaga, turnips, kohlrabi, radishes, cauliflower, African cassava, millet, babassu (a palm-tree coconut fruit popular in Brazil and Africa), cabbage and kale

- You are over 60

http://www.thyroid-info.com/hair

- You are in a period of hormonal change, such as perimenopause, menopause, pregnancy or post-partum

- You have had serious trauma to the neck, such as whiplash from a car accident or a broken neck

Symptoms

Common Hashimoto's/hypothyroidism symptoms that typically signal an underactive thyroid include:

- Hair loss
- Fatigue, exhaustion
- Depression, moodiness, sadness, difficulty concentrating, difficulty remembering
- Sensitivity to cold, cold hands and feet
- Inappropriate weight gain, or difficulty losing weight
- Dry, tangled or coarse hair
- Loss of hair from the outer part of the eyebrow
- Brittle fingernails
- Muscle and joint pains and aches
- Tendinitis in arms and legs, carpal tunnel syndrome
- Plantars fascitis - pain in the sole of the foot
- Swelling or puffiness in the eyes, face, arms or legs
- Heart palpitations
- Low sex drive
- Infertility, recurrent miscarriages
- Heavy, longer, more frequent or more painful menstrual periods
- High cholesterol levels, especially when it's unresponsive to diet and medication
- Worsening allergies, itching, prickly hot skin, rashes, hives (urticaria)
- Chronic infections, including yeast infections, oral fungus, thrush, and sinus infections
- Shortness of breath, difficulty drawing a full breath
- Constipation
- Full or sensitive feeling in the neck
- Raspy, hoarse voice

Common Graves' disease/hyperthyroidism symptoms, evidence of an overactive thyroid, include:

- Hair loss
- Rapid weight loss, or increased appetite without weight gain
- Insomnia, difficulty falling asleep or staying asleep
- Anxiety, erratic behavior, nervousness, irritability, nervousness, or panic attacks
- Difficulty concentrating, short attention span
- Palpitations, irregular heartbeat, high pulse and heartbeat
- Atrial fibrillation
- Feeling hot, sweating more than usual
- Hand tremors
- Diarrhea
- Fatigue
- Dry skin, thickened patches on shins and legs
- Fine, brittle hair
- Infertility
- Periods are lighter, less frequent, or stop altogether
- Muscle weakness, especially in the upper arms and thighs
- Eye problems, including double vision, scratchy eyes, bulging, sensitivity to light

Diagnosis

One self-test you can do to potentially detect some thyroid abnormalities is a thyroid neck check. To take this self-test, hold a mirror so that you can see the area of your neck just below the Adam's apple and right above the collarbone. This is the general location of your thyroid gland.

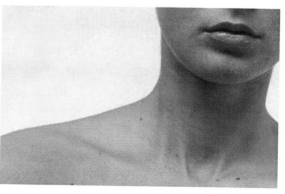

Tip your head back, while keeping this view of your neck and thyroid area in your mirror. Take a drink of water and swallow. As you swallow, look at your neck. Watch carefully for any bulges, enlargement, protrusions, or unusual appearances in this area when you swallow. Repeat this process several times.

If you see any bulges, protrusions, lumps or anything that appears unusual, see your doctor right away. You may have an enlarged thyroid, or a thyroid nodule, and your thyroid should be evaluated. Be sure you don't get your Adam's apple confused with your thyroid gland. The Adam's apple is at the front of your neck, the thyroid is further down, and closer to your collarbone.

NOTE: Remember that this test is by no means conclusive, and can't rule out thyroid abnormalities. It's just helpful to identify a particularly enlarged thyroid or masses in the thyroid that warrant evaluation.

Another possible sign of thyroid abnormality is a low basal body temperature. Some practitioners even believe that a low basal body temperature (taken upon awakening, in bed, before getting up and before any substantial movement) can be indicative of hypothyroidism. Typically, basal body temperatures lower than 97.8 to 98.2 degrees Fahrenheit are thought to potentially indicate hypothyroidism. This self-testing method was popularized by the late Dr. Broda Barnes. Again, this test is not considered conclusive by many practitioners, and doesn't definitively diagnose or rule out thyroid abnormalities.

Blood tests are another key way of identifying thyroid problems. The most commonly performed test is the thyroid stimulating hormone (TSH) test. While ranges vary from lab to lab, the general "normal" range for TSH tests is from approximately .3 to 3.0 -- levels above 3.0

are evidence of hypothyroidism, and levels below .3 are indicative of hyperthyroidism. If your doctor runs a TSH test (also known as a serum thyrotropin test), a number under .3 can indicate possible hyperthyroidism. Over 3.0 is considered indicative of hypothyroidism.

> **Most laboratories, and many doctors, are still using the older TSH normal range of .5 to 5.0. Don't accept "normal" as a TSH test result. Ask for the actual number. And if your doctor thinks that a TSH above 3.0 is normal and won't treat you, find another doctor.**

Note: increasing numbers of doctors are finding that a TSH of around 1 - 2 is optimal for most people to feel well and avoid having hypothyroid or hyperthyroid symptoms.

There are a number of other blood tests that may be done to help diagnose hypothyroidism, including Total T4, Free T4, Total T3, Free T3, Antithyroid Antibodies and Anti Thyroid Peroxidase (Anti-TPO) Antibodies. The antibodies tests can detect the antibodies that signal the presence of Hashimoto's or Graves' disease, even when TSH levels are normal.

Diagnosis of thyroid disease can be difficult, particularly when you have borderline thyroid conditions, or when antibodies are present and causing symptoms, but bloodwork has yet to reflect the abnormalities. There are practitioners who believe that you do not need to have an elevated TSH level in order to actually be diagnosed and treated for hypothyroidism. Increasingly, innovative doctors are also viewing high-normal or normal TSH levels as possible evidence of low-level hypothyroidism.

Hair brings one's self-image into focus; it is vanity's proving ground. Hair is terribly personal, a tangle of mysterious prejudices.
~ Shana Alexander

If you can't get a thyroid test from your doctor, HealthCheckUSA offers online and telephone ordering of three different test options: a standard TSH test; the Comprehensive Thyroid Profile, which includes T3 Uptake, T4 Total, T7, and TSH; and Comprehensive Thyroid Profile II, which includes T3 (Triiodothyronine) Free, T4 (Thyroxine) free, and TSH. The tests are priced extremely affordably, and HealthCheckUSA doctors sign off on bloodwork requests, and you receive the results directly, online, or by mail. You can order tests by calling 1-800-929-2044 or by visiting the web site at http://www.healthcheckusa.com

Ultimately, what is required is a complete clinical evaluation of your thyroid, involving an examination of the thyroid by a professional, who will feel for enlargement, nodules and masses. Your reflexes will be checked -- sluggish reflexes can be a sign of hypothyroidism, and hyperresponsive reflexes are more common in hyperthyroidism. Other clinical details will be observed, and family history discussed.

The clinical observation, in combination with symptoms, plus the results of blood tests should all be taken together to enable diagnosis of thyroid disease.

Graves' Disease/Hyperthyroidism Treatment

If you have a milder case of Graves' disease/hyperthyroidism, your doctor may initially prescribe antithyroid drugs such as methimazole (Tapazole) or propylthiouracil (PTU), as these drugs offer some chance of a remission. Despite the fact that as many as 40% of patients treated with antithyroid drugs can achieve a permanent remission, radioactive iodine (RAI) treatment is, however, the treatment of choice in the U.S., while antithyroid drugs are the primary treatment in other countries. By partially or fully disabling the thyroid, RAI eliminates hormone overproduction. Mot people who receive RAI become hypothyroid, and require lifelong thyroid hormone replacement.

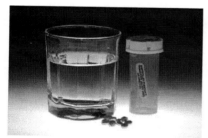

Some innovative practitioners recommend a technique known as block replace therapy (BRT), which involves simultaneous use of antithyroid drugs to disable the overproduction, and thyroid hormone replacement to suppress function and provide sufficient thyroid hormone.

Surgery, known as thyroidectomy, is typically done when you cannot tolerate antithyroid drugs, or are not a good candidate for RAI (such as in a case of life-threatening hyperthyroidism during pregnancy).

Thyroid Cancer

The treatment for thyroid cancer is typically surgical removal of the thyroid, followed by radioactive iodine to ablate any remaining thyroid tissue. Ultimately, without a functional thyroid, lifelong hypothyroidism sets in, and requires thyroid hormone replacement therapy.

Nodules/Goiter

The treatment for nodules is thyroid hormone replacement to suppress nodule growth. In some cases, ethanol injections or ultrasound may be used to remove the nodules. If nodules are suspected to be cancerous, or become large, cosmetically unsightly, or interfere with breathing or swallowing, the nodules – or the entire gland -- may be surgically removed.

In goiter – an enlarged thyroid -- the treatment is thyroid hormone replacement to suppress thyroid growth. If the gland become large, cosmetically unsightly, or interferes with breathing or swallowing, the gland may be surgically removed.

In either case, if all or part of the thyroid is removed, lifelong hypothyroidism may set in, requiring thyroid hormone replacement therapy.

Thyroid Hormone Replacement Therapy / Treating Hypothyroidism

Ultimately, most thyroid conditions – Graves' disease, hyperthyroidism, thyroid nodules, thyroid cancer, goiter, Hashimoto's disease – result in a person being hypothyroid, with an underactive, inactive, or surgically-removed thyroid.

Conventional treatment for hypothyroidism is with prescription thyroid hormone replacement drugs, almost always taken daily. Options are summarized in the chart on the following page.

Most commonly, a levothyroxine (T4) drug is prescribed, as this is considered the "standard" treatment for hypothyroidism. The most popular levothyroxine drug with physicians is Synthroid.

The term "Synthroid" is sometimes used interchangeably with "thyroid hormone replacement drugs," much in the same way that the brand name Kleenex has, for example, become synonymous with "tissue."

THYROID HORMONE REPLACEMENT DRUGS

GENERIC NAME	BRAND NAME	DESCRIPTION
Levothyroxine (Synthetic T4)	Synthroid, Levoxyl, Unithroid, Levothroid	The most common treatment, provides synthetic version of one hormone, T4. Different brands may have different fillers, dyes and potential allergens.
Liothyronine (Synthetic T3)	Cytomel	T3 drug that is often given with levothyroxine
Liotrix (Synthetic T4 + T3)	Thyrolar	A combination synthetic drug
Time-released, compounded T4 and/or T3	No brands	Currently available only from compounding pharmacies
Natural, desiccated thyroid	Armour Thyroid, Naturethroid	Derived from thyroid gland of pigs, includes T4, T3 and other thyroid hormones including T1 and T2

The popularity of Synthroid is mainly due to extensive marketing by the manufacturer, however, and all the brands of levothyroxine are considered to be similar in quality, potency and effectiveness.

Research and clinical practice of many thyroid experts has shown, however, that some patients feel better only with the addition of T3, and so increasing numbers of practitioners are prescribing levothyroxine plus liothyronine (Cytomel), a synthetic T4 plus T3 combination drug known as liotrix (Thyrolar), or less commonly, levothyroxine plus compounded T3.

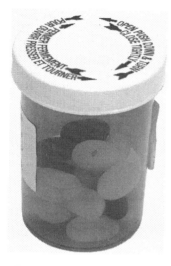

From the early 1900s until the 1950s, the only form of thyroid replacement drug available was natural, desiccated thyroid, namely, Armour Thyroid. The drug fell out of favor with some endocrinologists, as Synthroid's extensive marketing sold synthetic thyroid as a better, more modern option for thyroid treatment in the second half of the 20th century.

Marketing efforts aside, since the 1990s, Armour Thyroid has been enjoying a resurgence in popularity with some patients and practitioners. Derived from the dried thyroid gland of pigs, the drug contains natural forms of numerous thyroid hormones and nutrients typically found in an actual thyroid gland. Some patients report improvement in symptoms using natural thyroid, versus the synthetic options.

OPTIMIZING YOUR THYROID TREATMENT

If after treatment, you are still suffering from thyroid symptoms, including hair loss, there's a good chance that your thyroid treatment is not optimized.

http://www.thyroid-info.com/hair

Page 51

If you're on levothyroxine, make sure that you're on the right brand.

Some people do better on Synthroid, others on Levoxyl, or Levothroid. Stick with a brand name, however, and not a generic, to ensure consistency, because every time you refill a generic prescription, you can get a different manufacturer's product, and the potential for different potency.

Ask for additional T3 if it's needed.

Some people do not feel their best, and continue losing hair, unless their treatment also includes a second thyroid hormone, known as T3. T3 is the active thyroid hormone.

While it's a controversial topic that is under increasing study by various experts, some physicians do believe that supplemental T3 may be a solution to help optimize thyroid treatment for some patients. They add T3 in one of several ways:

- Added to levothyroxine treatment, via the addition of the prescription T3 drug Cytomel.
- Compounded time-released T3 in addition to levothyroxine
- Combination synthetic drug Thyrolar, which includes both T4 and T3
- Natural desiccated thyroid, such as the prescription drug Armour Thyroid, which also includes a full array of natural thyroid hormones, including T3

Consider natural thyroid.

Some practitioners believe that certain patients simply do best on natural desiccated thyroid, derived from the thyroid gland of pigs. These products, including Armour and Nature-throid, are prescription thyroid drugs. Keep in mind that many conventional physicians feel that these drugs are "out of date" and won't prescribe them, so you may need to find an open-minded doctor, or a holistic or alternative physician, in order to take these drugs.

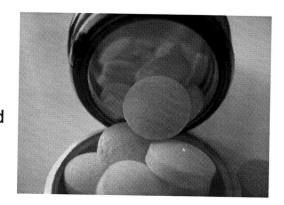

Take your medication properly.

There are a number of guidelines on how to properly take thyroid hormone, to ensure that you are absorbing the drug and receiving the maximum possible benefit.

- Don't take your thyroid hormone replacement drug within four hours of taking calcium supplements, or calcium-fortified juice. The same rule applies for antacids -- like Tums, or Mylanta in liquid or tablet form – which also contain calcium and can delay or reduce the absorption of your thyroid hormone.

- Don't take thyroid hormone replacement drugs within four hours of taking any supplements that contain iron, including prenatal vitamins, which usually are high in iron.

THYROID GUIDE TO HAIR LOSS

- Try to take your thyroid hormone around the same time each day. For best results, maximum absorption, and minimum interference from food, fiber and supplements, doctors recommend taking it in the morning on an empty stomach, about an hour before eating. New studies, however, have shown that taking your thyroid medication at bedtime (making sure that there are a few hours since you've eaten dinner) may result in even better absorption.

- If you need to take your thyroid hormone with food, be consistent and always take it with food. Don't switch back and forth between taking it with and without food.

- If you start or stop a high-fiber diet, or the diet drug Xenical/Alli (orlistat) while you are on thyroid hormone, have your thyroid function retested around six to eight weeks after your dietary change. High-fiber diets, and fat-absorbing medications can change the speed of thyroid drug absorption, and you may require a dosage adjustment. You should also be consistent about your daily fiber intake. Don't have 10 grams one day, and 30 grams the next day, and so on, or you're risking erratic absorption.

- If you are taking the Levoxyl brand of levothyroxine, take the drug with enough water and swallow the pill quickly. The pill dissolves rapidly, and if it dissolves in your mouth before swallowing it, you risk not absorbing all of the active ingredients.

THYROID GUIDE TO HAIR LOSS

Ensure you're getting proper nutrition for thyroid function.

You'll want to make sure that you're getting sufficient nutrition. Some recommendations, which are discussed at length in my book *Living Well With Hypothyroidism*, include:

- Take a high-potency multivitamin (note: if you're iodine sensitive, some vitamins come without iodine)
- Take a probiotic supplement that puts "good" bacteria into your digestive system
- Take supplemental zinc, which is important for thyroid hormone production and conversion
- Take supplemental selenium, which can help with conversion of T4 to T3, and may modulate autoimmunity.
- Take l-tyrosine, an amino-acid precursor to thyroid hormone
- Take z-guggulsterone -- known as "guggul" – an Ayurvedic remedy that is thyroid-stimulating
- Take essential fatty acid (EFA) supplements (because EFAs cannot be produced in the body)

Consider other ways to improve thyroid function.

- Minimize your intake of raw goitrogens: the foods that promote formation of goiters, and can act to slow down the thyroid. Some popular goitrogens include broccoli, brussels sprouts, cabbage, cauliflower, kales, soy products, and turnips.

- Reduce toxic exposures : reduce exposure to fluoride, perchlorate, and mercury – some of the toxins thought to negatively affect the thyroid
- Treat chronic infections, including gingivitis, *yersinia*, candida, and other bacterial infections
- Practice yoga, including specific shoulderstand poses that benefit the thyroid

GETTING A GREAT THYROID DOCTOR IS CRITICAL

The specialty for thyroid disease is endocrinology. Endocrinologists are doctors who specialize in diseases of the endocrine system. Endocrinologists typically have the initials F.A.C.E., after their names, standing for Fellow, American College of Endocrinology. The two main issues endocrinologists typically deal with are diabetes and thyroid problems. Some endocrinologists, however, have sub-specialties like reproductive endocrinology (fertility), nuclear medicine, growth disorders, or osteoporosis.

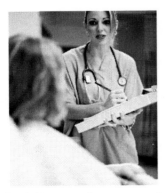 Most endocrinologists, however, focus on treating diabetes – not thyroid disease -- and aren't prepared for the difficulties and complexities of diagnosing and managing the typical thyroid patients, or their post-treatment symptoms.

Internists and general practice doctors sometimes provide decent diagnosis and ongoing treatment of thyroid disease, but the quality of thyroid care is hit or miss – and depends on the individual's knowledge and experience with thyroid patients.

When you are having difficulty getting diagnosed, or you don't do well on the conventional approach, or when you want to understand more about the many side effects and symptoms of hypothyroidism, the fairly conventional focus of most internists and general practice doctors may fall short of what you need.

That's when you should consider an osteopathic, holistic or metabolically-oriented physician with expertise in thyroid disease, metabolism, and hormonal medicine.

Unfortunately, many doctors -- whether general practitioners, primary care doctors, endocrinologists, ob-gyns, or others, believe the overly simplified conventional view of thyroid disease. They think it's easy to diagnose, and easy to treat, and *that it doesn't have anything to do with your hair loss.*

If you are struggling with a doctor like this – one who refuses to test your thyroid, or doesn't take your symptoms into account, then visit my **Thyroid Top Doctors Directory** at **http://www.thyroid-info.com/topdrs**

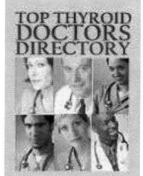

The **free** directory features patient recommended practitioners around the nation and around the globe, organized by state or country, along with comments by practitioners. It's a terrific resource, by patients, for patients, that can help you find just the right practitioner.

SECTION 3
HAIR LOSS TREATMENTS

As we have seen, hair loss can have a profound affect on an individual's self-esteem. Historically, there have always been remedies for hair loss and in our day and age, there are more than ever. The hair growth and remedy industry is a multi-billion dollar concern that keeps on growing – both in terms of good research and the next new fraud. Because making hair makes so much money, it is important for you, the consumer, to have an understanding of what might work before you invest both your money and your emotions. We'll take a tour through the options that are currently available and also look at what might be coming in the future.

DRUG TREATMENTS (ORAL AND TOPICAL)

Corticosteroids

Corticosteroids – "steroids" -- are sometimes used in the treatment of AA. Corticosteroids are drugs that mimic the hormone cortisol, which is produced by the adrenal glands. Cortisol and corticosteroids "suppress" the body's immune system, and prevent the errant immune cells from attacking hair follicles. Steroid drugs may be injected into the patchy spots affected by AA, taken orally or administered topically as an ointment or cream.

Given the painful nature of injections, topical corticosteroid ointments are often given to children; they are, however, considered less effective. Results vary, and are not universal. Some people respond; others have no change.

Corticosteroids are powerful drugs, however, and can cause undesirable side effects in some patients, including increased appetite, weight gain, headache, mood swings, sleeping difficulty, blood sugar fluctuations, and elevated cholesterol, among many other side effects.

Minoxidil (Rogaine)

Rogaine Another drug that is used is minoxidil (also known by its brand name, Rogaine.) A 5% topical solution is used to promote hair growth and may be used in adults and children when treating AA. Applied twice daily, new hair growth may appear in about 12 weeks.

In terms of treatment, minoxidil (Rogaine) is known to prolong the anagen (growing) stage of the hair cycle, but its effectiveness in offsetting the effects of stress hormones is unknown. It is clear that for individuals suffering from TE, comprehensive management of symptoms and underlying factors, such as nutritional deficiencies, should be considered. Non-pharmacological options such as counseling and mind-body approaches for stress and anxiety reduction may also be useful. Acute TE generally resolves without medical treatment or intervention.

Minoxidil is an FDA-approved, topically applied remedy for hair loss that is now available without a prescription. Though it may be less effective than when used by men, minoxidil is currently the only hair loss remedy that is approved for use by women. Minoxidil is best utilized for general thinning on the top of their head.

**When others kid me about being bald,
I simply tell them that the way I figure it,
the good Lord only gave men so many hormones,
and if others want to waste theirs on growing hair,
that's up to them.**
~ John Glenn

Minoxidil is a vasodilator and was originally developed for use as a medication for high blood pressure. Although the mechanism by which minoxidil works is not completely known, it appears to enlarge hair follicles that have become miniaturized, prolong the anagen phase of hair growth and cause some non-producing follicles to again enter the anagen phase. Hair that is regrown using minoxidil is usually on the top of the head, not the hairline and has a finer, softer texture than original terminal hairs. Varying studies report that hair regrowth may be seen in 10 to 20% of individuals using it while hair loss is slowed in approximately 90% of those using it. Minoxidil appears to be more effective in younger men who have not lost most of their hair.

Minoxidil must be applied twice a day to the scalp for at least four months before results are seen. Application of the product must continue indefinitely, as hair that is grown with the medication will be lost when use of the product is stopped. The long term effects of using the product are not known but the positive effects – regrowth and reducing hair loss may fade over time and with age. As noted, minoxidil is available in two dosages. Although the 5% product appears to be more effective, in women it may cause increased facial and ear hair if the topical medication leaves the scalp area.

Common side effects include itching and redness of scalp. Side effects that are cause for concern include dizziness, increased heart rate, weight gain and swelling of hands or feet. Complaints about using the solution include a greasy feeling to the scalp and the annoyance of applying twice daily on an ongoing basis. Minoxidil is sometimes used in combination with the prescription drug Retin-A (tretinoin) which is used topically for acne. Tretinoin irritates skin cells, causing a more rapid turnover in cells. It is unclear whether this combination is effective.

Given that, minoxidil may be a good product to try for the regrowth of hair on the top of the scalp.

Finasteride (Propecia)

Finasteride was originally developed and marketed as the drug "Proscar." Proscar is a drug prescribed for treatment of 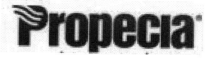 benign prostate hyperplasia (enlargement of the prostate gland). Under the brand name "Propecia," finasteride 1% is available by prescription only as an FDA approved oral treatment for androgenetic alopecia. Finasteride decreases the level of DHT circulating in the blood. Over time, this decrease in DHT causes a reduction in the miniaturization and cessation of follicle function found in androgenetic alopecia.

Like minoxidil, Propecia is best suited for younger men who have not yet experienced significant hair loss. For men who are balding, a prescription for Propecia is often combined with use of minoxidil. Propecia is not approved for use by women of child-bearing age due to the highly increased possibility of fetal birth defects. Women are discouraged from even handling the pills. The use of Propecia for women remains controversial elsewhere although a very small study (five women) in Switzerland found that postmenopausal women who ingested 2.5 mg per day of finasteride experienced a decrease in hair loss, an increase in hair growth and an improved appearance of their hair.

Different studies have shown varying results for men who used finasteride to treat androgenetic alopecia - 50 – 60% of men using it regrew hair on their scalp and one study showed that finasteride stopped hair loss in 91% of male patients. For some men, however, the drug did not reverse or slow their hair loss.

Side effects when taking finasteride are experienced by approximately 2 – 5% of men taking the drug. Again, given its involvement with hormones, the most common side effects of taking finasteride are related to sexual function - reduction in sexual drive, decrease in semen quantity and impotency that is reversible upon cessation of treatment. A small 2002 study found circumstantial evidence that mild to severe depression developed in patients taking finasteride. The Propecia website lists other possible side effects including rash, itching, hives, facial swelling, problems with ejaculation, breast tenderness and enlargement and testicular pain.

Like minoxidil, finasteride can be expensive over the long term, may take up to six-months to a year for results and must be continued for regrowth to be maintained. As well, the long term effects of taking finasteride are not known. Given its androgen blocking ability, finasteride may also lower PSA test results so inform your doctor if you are using it. Minoxidil and finasteride are the only two FDA approved medications for treatment of androgenetic alopecia.

Dutasteride (Avodart)

Dutasteride is a prescription drug developed to treat disorders of the prostate gland. It is a 5-alpha reductase inhibitor and thus blocks some of the effect of DHT in hair follicles. It is taken orally and when used off-label for hair loss, it may reduce the amount of hair that is lost. Like other compounds that affect androgen activity, side effects include decrease in libido, difficulty ejaculating, breast tenderness or enlargement and impotence. As well, dutasteride may remain in the body for months after use of the drug has been stopped. This means side effects or adverse reactions to the medication may take a very long time to resolve. Again, there is a lack of targeted studies proving that this drug's benefits outweigh the concerns.

Anthralin (Psoriatec)

Anthralin, a synthetic tar-like substance that alters immune function in the affected skin, is an approved treatment for psoriasis. Anthralin is also commonly used to treat alopecia areata. Anthralin is applied for 20 to 60 minutes ("short contact therapy") to avoid skin irritation, which is not needed for the drug to work. When it works, new hair growth is usually evident in 8 to 12 weeks. Anthralin is often used in

Page 63

combination with other treatments, such as corticosteroid injections or minoxidil, for improved results.

Sulfasalazine

A sulfa drug, sulfasalazine has been used as a treatment for various autoimmune disorders, including psoriasis. It acts on the immune system and has been used in patients with severe alopecia areata.

Topical Sensitizers

Topical sensitizers are medications that, when applied to the scalp, provoke an allergic reaction that leads to itching, scaling, and eventually hair growth. If the medication works, new hair growth is usually established in 3 to 12 months. Two topical sensitizers are used in alopecia areata: squaric acid dibutyl ester (SADBE) and diphenylcyclopropenone (DPCP). Their safety and consistency of formula are currently under review.

Oral Cyclosporine

Originally developed to keep people's immune systems from rejecting transplanted organs, oral cyclosporine is sometimes used to suppress the immune system response in psoriasis and other immune-mediated skin conditions. But suppressing the immune system can also cause problems, including an increased risk of serious infection and possibly skin cancer. Although oral cyclosporine may regrow hair in alopecia areata, it does not turn the disease off. Most doctors feel the dangers of the drug outweigh its benefits for alopecia areata.

Cimetidine (Tagamet)

Cimetidine is used to treat gastro-intestinal disorders such as ulcers

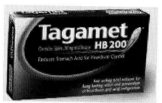

and reflux. It is available by prescription and over-the-counter and is taken in oral form. Cimetidine is thought to have a weak anti-androgen effect but no studies to date establish its use as a hair loss remedy. Side effects include impotence, loss of libido, nervousness and hallucinations.

Cyproterone Acetate (Diane-35)

Cyproterone acetate is a prescription anti-androgen that is not available in the United States. Used in Europe for treatment of prostate gland enlargement, cyproterone blocks the binding of DHT at receptor sites in the prostate and hair follicle. Drug studies on this medicine are conflicting and side effects include weight gain, depression and menstrual irregularities. (Given the potential for birth defects, this drug should not be used by women who anticipate becoming pregnant.)

Flutamide (Eulexin)

Flutamide (brand name Eulexin) is another prescription drug that was developed to treat disorders of the prostate gland. It is a nonsteroidal anti-androgen, taken orally, that binds up DHT receptors in the prostate and elsewhere. Because of its anti-androgen effect, it is also sometimes prescribed to slow hair loss. As with other prescription drugs that are prescribed off-label for hair loss – meaning that the drug's primary function is not to treat hair loss -- there are no large scale studies that show that these drugs will produce cosmetically acceptable results. Flutamide can cause liver failure and individuals choosing to use flutamide should be sure to be monitored regularly while using this drug. Other side effects include decreased fertility, hot flashes, breast tenderness or enlargement in men and women as well as a number of other symptoms. Read your patient pamphlet carefully if you use this drug.

Oral Contraceptives

Oral contraceptives (OCP) – birth control pills -- are often prescribed for women suffering from androgenetic alopecia. Because OCP's regulate hormone levels, OCP's might be useful for women whose bodies produce too many androgen hormones. OCP's are sometimes combined with other drugs, such as spironolactone, minoxidil or flutamide. Obviously, women with concerns for their fertility should not use these drugs for at least four to six months before trying to get pregnant as they may cause birth defects.

Spironolactone (Aldactone)

Spironolactone (brand name: Aldactone) is a prescription drug that is an aldosterone receptor antagonist, that is, it is used for people whose bodies produce too much of a hormone known as aldosterone. It is used to treat high blood pressure and fluid retention caused by heart, liver or kidney disease. Because it does have an effect on circulating hormones, it is also used as an anti-androgen to reduce (by blocking) high levels of DHT that are thought to be a primary cause of androgenetic alopecia.

Spironolactone is a powerful drug with many side effects. As it does alter hormones, it may cause unwelcome side effects in men such as reduction in sexual drive, decrease in semen quantity and impotency that is reversible upon cessation of treatment. In women it can cause irregular menstrual periods, post-menopausal vaginal bleeding and deepening of voice as well as enlarged or tender breasts in both men and women. Because it is a diuretic, it is recommended that it be taken in early in the day.

When used for hair loss, spironolactone helps reduce the rate of hair loss, but it has not shown to be effective for hair regrowth in women.

Photochemotherapy / Psoralen and Ultraviolet Radiation (PUVA) Treatment

In photochemotherapy, a treatment used most commonly for psoriasis, a person is given a light-sensitive drug called Psoralen either orally or topically and then exposed to an ultraviolet (UVA) light source. This combined treatment is called PUVA, or sometimes *Psoralen photo chemotherapy.*

Patients must go to a treatment center where the equipment is available at least two to three times per week. In clinical trials, approximately 55 percent of people achieve cosmetically acceptable hair growth using photochemotherapy. However, the relapse rate is high, and it's estimated that the rate of relapse after successful response to PUVA is 30% to 50%.. PUVA can cause headache, dizziness, a sunburn-like irritation, nausea, itching or stinging in the skin.

http://www.thyroid-info.com/hair
© 2008 Mary J. Shomon. All Rights Reserved

Page 67

Furthermore, the treatment carries the risk of developing skin cancer, including squamous cell carcinoma, basal cell carcinoma and the most dangerous form, malignant melanoma.

HAIR CARE/HAIR LOSS PRODUCTS

There are any number of hair product lines and tools specifically formulated to address hair loss. Many have unclear claims, a marked absence of references to actual research or legitimate studies, and sometimes confusing ingredient lists. Most offer shampoo, conditioner, "revitalizers" and a dietary supplement. Most are expensive. Some products have money-back guarantees that are not always honored.

Many of these hair loss remedies and supplements depend upon the consumer to believe the simple adage that "if some is good, more is better." That is, if iron, or certain amino acids, minerals or the chemical factors of certain herbs are present in a well-balanced diet – then more of them must be better if you are losing your hair.

One thing to be savvy about with regard to hair loss products is "the next greatest thing." Miracle drugs, amazing claims, revitalizers – like buses, there will be another hair loss remedy along in a few minutes.

Consider the story of a product called "Folliguard," that consisted of shampoo, pills and a "topical activator" at a cost of about $350. Promoters of the drug claimed that the product was "revolutionary" and "proven to rejuvenate hair in 90% of people who use it." Although Folliguard contained minoxidil, a nonprescription drug that has shown to be effective for hair loss, the Maine State Attorney

General sued its promoters in 2003 for representing their product to be unique and to provide guaranteed hair growth at a rapid rate. The defendants in the case settled the matter by promising not to falsely advertise their product and to pay penalties to customers and failing to honor their money-back guarantee.

Today you can purchase Avacor, another product with pills, hair care items and a guarantee. The cost of Avacor Men (or Women) is $499.95. Avacor's website lists the active ingredient for their "Topical Formulation" as minoxidil 5%. While minoxidil has been approved by the FDA for use as a hair loss treatment, it is available for a lot less at your local drugstore under the brand name "Rogaine." Caveat emptor – take a good, close look at any product you may contemplate purchasing. Look at the ingredients, then research the ingredients, ask your doctor, but don't rely upon Internet testimonials, or as in the case of Folliguard noted above, Internet guarantees.

Note: A good website to check out before buying any hair loss remedy is http://www.hairlossscams.com/index.html.

Aminexil / Kevis

Aminexil is a formula developed by Loreal that can be found in combination products with minoxidil. The product is claimed to prevent collagen formation around hair follicles and thus increase survival of the follicle. Larger studies using FDA standards are needed to verify the usefulness of Aminexil.

Another line that claims to prevent hair loss through scalp hygiene are the Kevis products that "address hair and scalp hygiene through the application of the biological compound, hyaluronic acid." The Kevis Extra Strength Hair and Scalp lotion appear to be water based but the website language claims that the active ingredient (ingredient lists not readily available on the website) works under the skin at the follicle level to "fill in DHT receptor" sites. Neither the prices for various products nor a money-back guarantee are apparent on the website.

HairMax Laser Comb

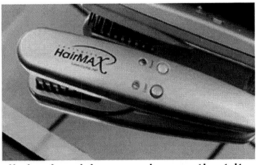

Lasers have been used for some years for the removal of unwanted hair. The HairMax Laser Comb claims to reduce hair loss and promote regrowth through the application of low-level laser light to the scalp. The FDA has approved the HairMax Laser Comb, and some clinical evidence shows that it may help with hair loss.

Illustrations on the HairMax website seem to indicate that application of laser light provides "energy" to the "hair growth process" thus improving hair texture and quantity. Other internet claims note that the HairMax Laser Comb increases blood supply to the hair follicle. Most hair loss isn't generally caused by a lack of blood supply to the scalp and follicle, it is caused by genetics, miniaturization of the hair follicle and the interaction of chemicals created in our bodies as we age. While minoxidil is a vasodilator, it also has an inhibitory effect on DHT in the hair follicle. There is no evidence that the Laser Comb does. However, it is one more treatment that may be worth trying.

The cost of the HairMax Laser Comb Premium is approximately $545.

Nizoral

Ketoconazole (brand name Nizoral) is an anti-fungal agent that is prescribed for systemic fungal infections such as oral thrush. It is also formulated in a shampoo for use in treating the scaling caused by dandruff and seborrheic dermatitis. As an anti-fungal, Nizoral may reduce topical inflammation of the scalp which may have an effect on hair loss (to the extent that inflammation is causing the hair loss). Larger studies on this effect are needed.

Phyto

Phyto is a hair products company that users botanical ingredients to create products for a variety of hair conditions including dry, frizzy, aging and thinning hair. The Phyto website indicates that their "decoctions work in synergy to ensure maximum results…" which, to the lay reader, appears to be the kind of hairspeak that should convince us that expensive hair care products are worth the money.

Of their hair loss line they note "these *Phyto* formulas purify, soothe, and care for the scalp to stimulate the hairbulb area and regenerate growth." While cleansing of the scalp is important, it is unlikely that any topical shampoo, conditioner or lotion can affect the "hairbulb" area – the "bulb" of the hair follicle is located under the skin. The primary ingredients in their formulations are also not known to "regenerate" hair growth. This sort of claim, while attractive, should be considered carefully.

Their dietary supplements to combat hair loss consist primarily of vitamin supplements and the energizing shampoo is formulated with ginseng and zinc. Although zinc may have future promise, there isn't sufficient evidence at this time to consider topical application of zinc will counter hair loss.

How can I control my life when I can't control my hair?
~ Anonymous

Nioxin

Another hair care line that utilizes a wealth of botanical, herbal and vitamin preparations is the Nioxin line. This line has eight "systems" each of which includes multiple products.

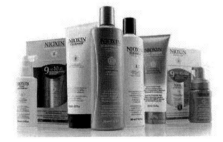

On the Nioxin website, language reads "a daily regimen of cleansing, moisturizing and nourishing, each NIOXIN system works to help improve the appearance of thinning hair and create and maintain an optimum scalp environment." Note here that the claim is to "improve the appearance" of hair not the amount of it.

This manufacturer claims to "remove DHT" from the hair by cleaning and "safeguard against DHT buildup on the scalp." The detrimental effect of DHT on the hair follicle, however, occurs beneath the scalp level, below which these products actually work. Use of these types of potentially expensive hair line products is not likely to damage your hair, but they are not likely to stop or slow hair loss either.

Polysorbate 80

Polyoxyethylene sorbitan monooleate (known as Polysorbate 80) is a yellowish liquid that is used as an emulsifier and surfactant. It is often used in ice cream to give it a firmer texture as it melts. It first came to prominence in the hair loss remedy known as the "Helsinki Formula," which was the subject of extensive litigation in the 1980's. Testimonials on the Web point to the ability of polysorbate 80 to "clean DHT from the hair follicle" and to "promote a histamine response that promotes regeneration" of the hair shaft.

These claims appear dubious and there do not seem to be credible studies that point to a positive use or mechanism by which polysorbate 80 could be considered a positive addition to a hair loss remedy. Both polysorbate 80 and polysorbate 60 are actually considered to be potential carcinogens as well.

Procerin and Provillus

Procerin is a combination product that includes 1500 mg. of saw palmetto berries, saw palmetto extract, zinc sulfate and pyroxidine among its ingredients. The formulation of another hair line product, Provillus is very similar. Both products rely upon saw palmetto.

Claims on the Procerin product website indicate that Procerin works faster than other products but it is unclear why. At a glance, since saw palmetto may have a similar effect in the body to the drug finasteride is possible that Procerin or Provillus may be effective for some individuals given the inclusion of saw palmetto. As noted elsewhere in this guide, zinc sulfate (zinc oxide in Provillus), but is not proven. Procerin also includes GLA which is discussed in this guide's section on Evening Primrose Oil.

Sephren

Sephren is a combination hair loss remedy for women from the same folks that bring us Procerin. Sephren does not include saw palmetto but offers B vitamins, magnesium and herbs in its dietary supplement. The dietary supplement includes para-amino benzoic acid (PABA), also a suspected carcinogen (hence its removal from many sunscreens). The Sephren topical serum includes essential oils (cedarwood, thyme, rosemary and lavender) in a mixture of carrier oils (jojoba, grapeseed). In 1998, a randomized, double-blind research study of patients with alopecia areata did find this same combination of oils to be effective in treating the condition.

ThymuSkin

ThymuSkin was originally made with calf thymus extract (the thymus is a gland in the chest that is involved with immune function). ThymuSkin claims to "clean out each follicle freeing it from accumulated oil, dirt, sebaceous matter, debris and other waste."

Tricosaccaride

The compound Tricosaccaride was developed by Foltene Laboratories. According to documentation on a Foltene laboratories website, Tricosaccaride is a "particular mixture of natural mucopolysaccharides."

Mucopolysaccharides or glycosaminoglycans are sugar chains that play a role in cellular reproduction and neuronal communication. The website notes that "the importance of their [mucopolysaccharides] presence in the hair follicle is not completely clear" but that the proprietary compound, Tricosaccaride, improves the condition of hair, promotes hair growth and prevents "hair fall." The website language indicates this is done by increasing the number of hairs in the anagen (growing) stage and decreasing the number of hairs in the telogen (resting) stage of the hair cycle.

Although Foltene Laboratories is apparently unsure of the importance of mucopolysaccharides in the hair cycle as noted above, they have apparently conducted "37 clinical trials on a total of 1297 subjects" to prove the effects of product (no studies cited). Further conflicting language reads that "Tricosaccaride does not penetrate the tissues surrounding the follicle and is proven to have no side effects: its action takes place only at the level of the hair follicle and the surface skin layer." Referring to the illustration of the hair shaft in the earlier section of this guide, you will see that the hair follicle is found below the surface of the skin, but the action of this product takes place only at the surface skin layer. For the discerning consumer, the promotion of this product should bring to mind points discussed earlier about amazing claims, absence of credible studies and conflicting explanations of how a product works.

Tricomin / Folligen

Tricomin is manufactured by ProCyte, a company that has been working with copper peptides for a number of years. ProCyte has developed several products utilizing specific copper peptide formulations such as Iamin, an FDA approved wound dressing, GrafCyte which is used after hair transplant surgery to speed the healing process and Tricomin, a hair loss line. In the body, copper is involved with collagen production and connective tissue health among other functions. High doses of other supplements such as zinc, vitamin C and iron can deplete copper in the body. The ProCyte website notes advantages of copper compounds as wound healing, strengthening of the hair shaft, increase in collagen activity and assisting in hair cycle regulation.

Folligen is another product that includes a copper peptide formulation in its product. Some of the Folligen products include essential oils, saw palmetto and a variety of herbs as well. Saw palmetto is considered an anti-androgen and the copper peptide formulations may have merit. Folligen is often used in combination with minoxidil by women.

Viviscal

Viviscal is a hair product line that seems to be formulated with vitamins and "cartiligeous marine extract." The studies cited on the website are old and the research is noted as "non-standard" in other papers critical of the finding that "special marine extracts and silica compounds" are effective against androgenetic alopecia.

NUTRITION, HERBS AND SUPPLEMENTS

Your body is a miraculous, living organism. It ferries you throughout your day, all the while repairing itself and meeting the demands that are placed on it over the course of a lifetime. The body has relatively well known nutritional needs – enough protein, fiber, vitamins, water, carbohydrate and the like. If you are deficient in a nutritional area, it is likely that your body will show the result of that deficiency. For example, individuals suffering from eating disorders are known to display symptoms such as hair loss as a result of poor nutritional uptake. Any condition, illness or personal behavior that results in a lessening of the body's ability to receive, absorb or use necessary nutrients will likely result in physical symptoms of a deficiency. Correction of that deficiency will generally reverse the tide.

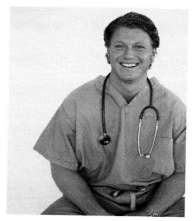

If you are actually deficient in a nutritional component necessary for the healthy production of hair, the quality and quantity of your hair will likely show it. Adding that component to your diet should, under normal circumstances, restore the appearance and amount of your hair.

Establishing whether you are nutritionally deficient requires blood tests. A qualified doctor or dermatologist can evaluate whether a nutritional deficiency may literally be at the root of your hair loss.

It is important to remember that all supplements, whether multi-vitamins, supplements or herbal preparations are medicines – they interact with your body chemistry in ways you may or may not know about. When visiting your doctor, always be sure to mention any supplements you are taking, not just prescription drugs.

In this section, you will read that there are not many large-scale, well-designed, unbiased reports that support the use of supplements for use as hair loss remedies. While this may seem discouraging for those who are looking for solid validation for their choices, it is true. As well, consumers should take note when evidence has been found that certain supplements can be dangerous or have been proven useless.

However, the lack of studies into a particular herb or vitamin does not necessarily mean that it may not be proven useful in the future – it simply means that well-considered data doesn't currently exist to validate that remedy. Within the dermatological industry, anecdotal value has been found for a number of "alternative" remedies, and calls for more thorough research will eventually be answered.

Evening Primrose Oil

Evening primrose (Oenothera biennis) is a North American wildflower with seeds that are ground for their oil and sold as capsule and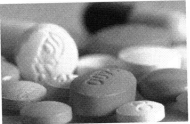

gelcaps. Used by Native Americans to speed healing of cuts and wounds, evening primrose oil ("EPO") contains essential fatty acids called linolenic acid ("LA"), as well as gamma-linolenic acid ("GLA"). Essential fatty acids are polyunsaturated fats (known as "PUFA's") that assist in metabolic regulation, brain function, physical growth and reproduction as well as skin and hair growth. They are called "essential" because they are not made by the body. The body can synthesize GLA from linolenic acid and it is later broken down into arachidonic acid. There are different types of PUFA's, including omega-3 and omega-6 fatty acids. LA, GLA and arachidonic acid are all omega-6 fatty acids.

Because it has anti-inflammatory effects, and may have an impact on the testosterone conversion process, EPO may prove beneficial for some hair loss.

B-Vitamins

B-vitamins are water-soluble and are important for a healthy body, where they assist with the synthesis of carbohydrates, breakdown of fats and proteins, health of skin and other systems. Of the eight B-vitamins, two B-vitamins are often mentioned with regard to hair loss, biotin and pyridoxine. Given the ease by which these vitamins are found in the North American diet (and the fact that biotin is manufactured within the intestine), deficiencies of either vitamin are not common. (Individuals who consume a high number of egg whites can, however, become deficient in biotin as egg whites contain a compound that binds with biotin.)

As we age, we may lose some of our ability to absorb B-vitamins from our diet and so B vitamin supplementation can be useful. A good-quality, high-potency B-complex vitamin can be a good source of these important vitamins.

DHEA

Dehydroepiandrosterone (DHEA) is a steroid hormone produced by the adrenal glands. When ingested as a supplement, DHEA can be

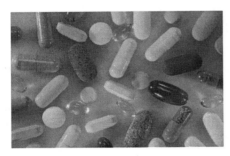

synthesized into androstenedione, testosterone, estrogen or other chemicals in the body. Despite extensive study, the role of DHEA (other than acting as a precursor for other hormones) remains unclear. Possibly because levels of DHEA decline with the aging process, DHEA is touted as "youth drug," or "anti-aging" pill – the thinking being that if DHEA levels are restored, so will youth (and lost hair). DHEA is an anabolic steroid it is still available as a nutritional supplement. You should not take DHEA unless you have had a DHEA-Sulfate (DHEA-S) test to evaluate whether or not you are deficient in DHEA.

Green Tea

Green tea (Camellia sinensis) has been used for centuries for a wide variety of health concerns. Green tea is made from unfermented leaves and purportedly contains a higher level of antioxidants, known as polyphenols, than other teas. Antioxidants forage for free radicals on a cellular level in the body. Free radicals are substances that damage cells, alter genetic material and can cause cell death.

Today green tea is widely consumed for pleasure and for its possible protective factors against a number of cancers and conditions such as heart disease. Individuals drinking green tea as a therapeutic agent should be cautious that it does not interfere with other supplements they are taking or physical conditions they may have.

Green tea is also considered to have an effect on circulating hormones in the blood. Individuals who consume higher levels of green tea have higher levels of a binding agent in their blood that attaches to hormones such as testosterone. This action is thought to have an effect on the synthesis of a 5-alpha reductase type I enzyme that is partly responsible for the formation of DHT (the powerful form of testosterone that is implicated in follicle death in androgenetic

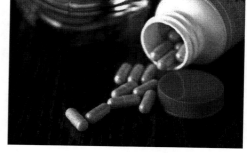

alopecia). Studies do not currently exist that explore the ability of green tea taken either orally or applied topically to reduce hair loss, but future studies may prove informative.

Iron

Iron is an essential trace element that is necessary for good health. It has many functions in the human body, including the transmission of oxygen in the blood, building of connective tissue, assisting in the composition of neurotransmitters in the brain as well as playing a role in the immune system. Some studies have suggested that iron deficiency may play a role in several types of alopecia.

Iron deficiency is characterized by a decline in red blood cell count and can be determined by a simple finger-prick test.

Lysine

Amino acids are the basic building blocks of proteins. Proteins are essential components of each cell in the body. There have been twenty amino acids identified, a number of which are essential, meaning they must be consumed. The best source of essential amino acids is protein such as meat, fish or eggs. One amino acid, lysine, is critical for the hair, yet is the most difficult amino acid to get enough of via diet. Lysine promotes the absorption of calcium, the production of enzymes and collagen for connective tissue and has a role in the immune system. A 2002 study notes that a deficiency of the l-lysine may play a role in hair loss.

A well-designed study found that supplementation with lysine and iron assisted in restoring hair in these cases. It's thought that when lysine and iron levels are low, the body switches some hair follicles off to increase levels elsewhere. Including lysine-rich foods and lysine supplements may be a help.

The tenderest spot in a man's make-up is sometimes the bald spot on top of his head
~ Helen Rowland

Arginine

L-arginine is also an amino acid and, among other functions, acts as precursor to the formation of nitrous oxide, a transitory substance in the body that assists in the maintenance of blood vessels, the immune system and beyond. Body builders have taken l-arginine supplements for years, trying to stimulate production of growth hormones to build musculature. Like lysine, arginine is found in meat, fish, nuts and eggs and it is also manufactured by the body.

Because both minoxidil and arginine are involved in action involving nitrous oxide, arginine is hoped to have a similar effect as minoxidil.

Methylsulfonylmethane (MSM)

Methylsulfonylmethane is a sulfur compound that occurs naturally in the body and is taken in from food as well. According to website claims, MSM assists with forming keratins, which are proteins that used to create fingernails, toenails and hair.

However, there are signaling pathways and enzymes that utilize MSM-like compounds to assist in transferring hormones in the blood and it is possible that there may be an as-yet unexplored effect there. There are no critical studies that support MSM for use as a hair-loss remedy.

As with so many other hair-loss treatments, time and self-experimentation may tell.

Saw Palmetto

Saw Palmetto (*Serenoa repens*), also known as American dwarf palm tree is an herbal product that appears to have an inhibitory effect on the conversion of testosterone to dihydrotestosterone. The ripe berries of the plant are dried, ground or used whole in a variety of forms such as capsules, liquid extract, or tea.

Saw Palmetto is used primarily to treat benign prostatic hyperplasia or BPH (commonly known as enlarged prostate). Although this would appear to be a similar affect on hair loss to that of that of the drug finasteride (Proscar, Propecia) there have not yet been sufficient independent studies in the United States to prove this herb is effective for the treatment of hair loss.

A small, industry funded study found that 60% of male study participants with androgenetic alopecia who received orally delivered botanical therapy, including saw palmetto, experienced some improvement in their condition. Another study found that saw palmetto extract compared well compared to finasteride and did not have as significant of an effect on sexual function.

Saw palmetto is widely used in Europe as a hair loss remedy and for treatment of BPH.

Pygeum / Beta-sitosterol

Pygeum (*Pygeum africanum)* is an evergreen tree found in Africa. It is known as an "African Plum" tree and the tree has become endangered due to the use of its bark to make medicinal teas and herbal compounds. The bark has traditionally been used for urinary tract disorders, stomach ache and even as an aphrodisiac by native Africans. Pygeum is widely used as an herbal remedy for prostate and urinary disorders in Europe but less so in the United States where use of saw palmetto is more common. Pygeum extract contains, among other things, phytosterols that might hinder the development of androgen precursors – thus blocking the synthesis of DHT.

Studies show that pygeum has good potential for use as a treatment for benign prostatic hyperplasia ("BPH"), but critical studies are lacking on whether pygeum would then be a worthwhile hair loss remedy. Side effects include mild stomach upset, nausea and diarrhea. Because of its possible hormonal action, pygeum is not recommended for women who are considering pregnancy.

It often appears that products that are used to treat BPH are then assumed to be appropriate treatments for hair loss. This assumption may have some basis in fact as androgenetic alopecia and BPH have similar hormonal signaling pathways. Another such preparation, beta-sitosterol, is made from plant materials such as Serenoa repens (saw palmetto) and Pygeum africanum (pygeum) among two. It contains phytosterols and is sometimes used for high cholesterol and to treat BPH in Europe. Again, as with other remedies available for sale, critical research doesn't support use of beta-sitostrol as a supplement to regrow hair. Further research may prove its appropriateness in that regard.

Zinc

As the 23rd most abundant element in the earth's crust, zinc is refined from zinc ore that is mined in more than fifty countries around the world. Zinc is utilized as coating to protect steel and iron, in the manufacture of precision components, in pharmaceuticals and cosmetics and as a micronutrient for plants, animals and humans. The U.S. Bureau of Mines estimates that an average person will use about 730 pounds of zinc in their lifetime. Zinc is an important mineral that the body uses to assist in regulating its cell division, wound healing, immune system and even the senses of taste and smell. Zinc is found in dairy products, brewer's yeast, meat, oysters and beans. Zinc deficiencies are generally found only in the undernourished or in developing countries.

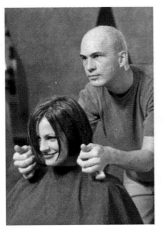

Zinc is found in a large number of hair loss products and remedies – supplements, shampoos, conditioners, treatments, etc. A form of zinc, zinc sulfate, has been found to have some effect on the synthesis of DHT (the deleterious form of testosterone that affects hair follicles). Zinc sulfate does not operate on the production of DHT directly, rather, it has a secondary function of reducing the effectiveness of a co-factor in the production of DHT. As zinc sulfate reduces the efficiency of NADPH, an electron carrier, it reduces the ease by which NADPH assists in the formation of DHT.

One 2002 study noted that there was no evidence to support the idea that low blood serum levels of zinc were a cause of hair loss. Anecdotally, however, zinc is considered important, and adding zinc as part of your diet, for example by adding dairy products or meat to your diet, or a low-dose supplement, may be helpful.

Nettles

The herbal treatment nettles (the herbal plant, Urtica dioica, also known as stinging nettle) is often recommended because of its properties as a potential DHT inhibitor.

Nettles has been used for prostate enlargement (BPH). Nettles functions both as a skin irritant, which have have beneficial properties for the skin, and it's thought that nettles may help block the enzymes that help convert testosterone to DHT

Some experts believe that, while studies have yet to be done, nettles might function like a weak version finasteride (Propecia). Use caution, however, and consult your doctor, as nettles is not recommended for anyone with heart disease, kidney problems, stomach problems, or allergic sensitivities.

ALTERNATIVE/HOLISTIC/INTEGRATIVE THERAPIES

Ayurvedic Medicine

Ayurvedic medicine is a practice from India that has developed over thousands of years of dialogue, experimentation and use. Ayurvedic practices seek to balance the physical and emotional energies of the individual. These holistic practices make use of lifestyle interventions as well as herbal preparations and treatments to balance the entire individual – as opposed to the more western philosophy of treating a particular condition or symptom. Ayurvedic medicine considers each person to have a particular constitution – "Vata," "Pitta" or "Kapha". Pitta individuals, or those who have too much Pitta in their system may be inclined to lose hair early or to have thinning hair. This sort of imbalance can be treated with meditation, herbal preparations, yoga, oil massage and other treatments.

A diet supplement for hair loss would include a "handful of white sesame seeds" every morning and some yogurt every day. Herbs that might be used for hair loss include dashamoola, bhringaraj and jatamamsi. An oil massage to increase blood circulation to the scalp could include bhringaraj oil or brahmi oil which is applied to the scalp regularly to stimulate hair growth. Massage of the shoulders, neck and scalp are also recommended for relaxation and to increase circulation.

Ayuvedic treatment requires recommendations from an experienced practitioner.

Chinese Medicine

In Chinese medicine, hair loss is thought to be caused by a blood and kidney deficiency – a deficiency that causes hair follicles to be undernourished in some way – through the aging process or an underlying medical condition.

One herb used in traditional Chinese medicine for the treatment of alopecia is an herb known as He Shou Wu that is made from the roots of a plant known commonly as Chinese Knotweed (*Polygonum multiflorum*). He Shou Wu is a common ingredient in Chinese medicinal preparations and is thought to "nourish blood." It is often used for preventing grey hair and alopecia and for boosting energy. He Shou Wu is an herb found in the Chinese medicine preparation Shou Wu Wan.

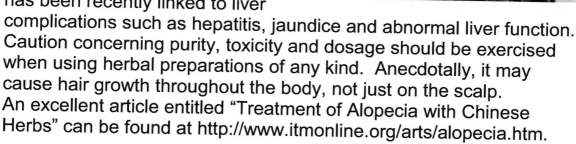

The herb contains compounds that may have antioxidant and anti-inflammatory effects in the body. Although He Shou Wu is known as being a relatively safe herb, it has been recently linked to liver complications such as hepatitis, jaundice and abnormal liver function. Caution concerning purity, toxicity and dosage should be exercised when using herbal preparations of any kind. Anecdotally, it may cause hair growth throughout the body, not just on the scalp. An excellent article entitled "Treatment of Alopecia with Chinese Herbs" can be found at http://www.itmonline.org/arts/alopecia.htm.

The article discusses the concepts of Chinese medicine with regard to alopecia and details ingredients of traditional tonics made for the prevention of hair loss.

Acupuncture

Acupuncture is a component of Chinese medicine that involves the use of thin needles through the skin at specific points on the body for relief of pain and other medical symptoms. Acupressure is a similar treatment that involves the application of pressure to specific points or meridians on the body.

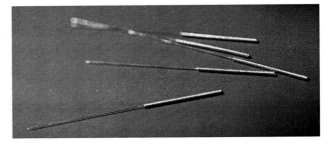

Anecdotal evidence exists for the use of acupuncture for the treatment of alopecia areata, but as noted above, since the course is not predictable, results cannot be precisely attributed to acupuncture. For those who use acupuncture and acupressure, the results are often relief of stress and increased energy. Stress is known to be an underlying cause and exacerbating factor in some forms of hair loss. While these treatments may not be widely advocated in the United States, they might be worth investigating to the extent that stress might be an underlying cause or result of hair loss.

Aromatherapy / Essential Oils

The use of plant parts for medicinal purposes is as old as mankind. Aromatherapy is an alternative medical practice that promotes the use of essential oils for better health and well being. Essential oils are concentrated extracts that are produced from many parts of botanical materials, such as the root, seeds, leaves, bark and flowers. Essential oils are often inhaled, diffused or applied topically. Like herbs, essential oils are used to treat a variety of ailments.

In a 1998 study, researchers using a randomized, double-blind study found that a combination of essential oils massaged into the scalp of 86 alopecia areata patients over a period of seven months resulted in an improvement in scalp hair in 44% of the active research group. By comparison, 15% of the control group experienced improvement during this period. Study participants massaged a combination of essential oils (thyme, rosemary, lavender and cedarwood, plus jojoba and grapeseed as carrier oils) into their scalp daily. The control group massaged only jojoba and grapeseed oils. The researchers who designed this study included the combination of cedarwood, lavender, thyme and rosemary because these particular essential oils have been historically promoted as a treatment for alopecia areata.

Essential oils are highly concentrated and can cause allergic skin reactions in some people. If you pursue the use of essential oils, consulting with an experienced and reputable practitioner for both advice and materials is advisable.

Topical Onion Juice

There is some evidence that topically applied onion juice can help treat alopecia areata. A study published in the *Journal of Dermatology* found that over six weeks, almost 90% of the people using the onion juice (as compared to only a small percentage using the control substance, water) had hair regrowth.

Biofeedback

Biofeedback is a method by which patients learn to control or observe their involuntary nervous system responses. Patients are given feedback on certain biological processes (galvanic skin resistance, skin temperature, heart rate, among others) to assist them with overcoming certain habits and for assistance in dealing with conditions or illnesses. For example, biofeedback exercises involving muscle tension can give a patient the ability to invoke a sense of relaxation in their body. Relaxation has been shown to have a positive effect on dermatological conditions that may have inflammation or anxiety as a trigger such as acne or psoriasis.

Hypnosis

Hypnosis has been found to boost the effectiveness of biofeedback exercises in dermatological patients. One study found that hypnosis can assist with or resolve the emotional and the psychological impact of conditions such as acne, alopecia areata and atopic dermatitis, among others. With regard to alopecia areata specifically, a small study found that use of hypnosis was able to significantly assist 28 patients with depression and anxiety they suffered over their condition. Approximately twelve of these patients also experienced regrowth of hair, however five individuals in the group also suffered hair loss.

Hypnotherapy has also been found to reduce the discomfort of some dermatological procedures as well. Research available at this time points to hypnosis as a good complementary treatment for individuals suffering emotional or psychological distress over any type of hair loss.

Cognitive Behavioral Methods/Stress Reduction

Cognitive behavior methods rely on replacing negative self-talk or behaviors with positive thoughts and behaviors. For this method, patient and therapist examine the methods of thought that are bothering a patient. By looking for triggers, such as "when I feel this...then I feel or think that" and identifying their negative influence, modes of thinking can be reframed and practiced that support a healthier emotional and physical view. This type of "thought substitution" can also influence dermatological conditions such as acne.

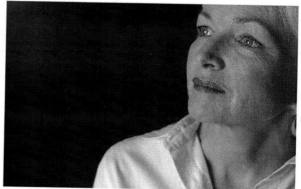

While large studies do not support these practices as "treatments" for hair loss, they are treatments for the stress that accompanies hair loss and significant stress by itself can be a cause of hair loss. The body is a complicated organism and stress plays a heavy role in disease throughout our lives. Most practices that induce a progressive sense of relaxation in the body will be helpful in reducing stress. Reduction of stress in the body is always helpful, whether one has hair loss or not.

But to the extent that hair loss may be exacerbated by stress, there are a number of well known avenues to explore including yoga, deep breathing, tai chi, imagery work and meditation. Any hobby or practice that you have, a daily walk, artwork or gardening - that gives you a sense of calm can give you a clue as to the types of things that can assist you in reducing your stress level. By replacing stress or anxious thinking with calming techniques and practices, you can positively affect your emotional outlook and physical well being.

HAIR REPLACEMENT PRODUCTS

Concealers

Concealers are products that mask patchy hair loss through a variety of means; creams, powders, lotions, sprays and fibers. Since concealers work on the concept of camouflage, they work best for thinning hair, not scalps that are predominantly bald. Concealers color the scalp, tone down scalp shine and can also add texture (through fibers or sprinkles) that fill in the thinning area.

Concealers are primarily made of emollients, which are products included in cosmetics to moisturize. Concealers can color and bulk up the shorter vellus hairs that occur with AGA, thus giving the appearance of a uniformly colored, fuller head of hair. They are often used in preparation for and after hair transplant surgery or in conjunction with minoxidil or Propecia.

Concealers are topical, they don't affect the hair follicle and they appear to be safe. Experimentation is key. Concealers are fast and relatively inexpensive for the appearance they provide. The downside of concealers is that they are temporary and can be messy. It is absolutely necessary to take the time to find a product that fits your needs. Practice when you have spare time in order to achieve the result that you desire.

Like cosmetics, concealers take time to apply. Some concealers can be worn while swimming, some not. All seem to be easily removed with shampoo. Again, take time to find the product that suits your needs. The most satisfied users of concealers seem to be those that are the most practiced at application. There are many hair loss blogs and forums on the internet where people are happy to give tips on brands and application methods. Concealers are a good temporary option for both men and women.

Products that seem to find approval with users of concealers include DermMatch Topical Shading (hard packed powder formula), Toppik (colored fibers that adhere to hair) and Couvre (camouflage lotion), among others.

Hair Extensions

Hair extensions are gaining popularity with both men and women. Hair extensions first came into the public eye via their use by celebrities who had short hair one day and long the next. While some of these styles are the result of clip-on extensions, many are created by the use of hair extensions that weave natural or synthetic hair onto existing hair. Hair weaves are now a common procedure for older women with hair that is thinning naturally or that have some underlying medical condition that has caused thinning or hair loss. Hair immediately looks thicker and fuller.

In a recent *New York Times* article, dermatologist Dr. Marc R. Avram noted that "with extensions, the positive is instant density...It's temporary, meaning you can take them out, it's a very good solution."

The process essentially involves bonding several pieces of hair to an existing hair relatively close to scalp level. Hair extensions are sold in bundles or in smaller sections called "wefts." The quality, color and texture of hair extensions vary widely. The most expensive extensions are those made from human hair. Extensions may be sold as "bonded" which means that the hair bundle is fused together at one end by an adhesive material. At the time of application, the adhesive end is placed on the natural hair and joined by a heating method or ultrasound.

Just as the quality and price of extensions varies, so does the experience of individuals applying extensions. When using extensions it is a good idea to find out if the person who will apply your extensions has been trained by the manufacturer of the extensions you have chosen to use. Ask for pictures of their work and references so that you may follow up with some of their clients. Don't be afraid to ask!

As hair extensions are essentially adding the weight of additional hair to one hair shaft, the added tension on the hair shaft can cause traction alopecia – the loss of hair due to undue stress on the hair follicle. While this condition may occur with even the best applied extensions, it happens more often with applications that are done poorly. A well done hair weave should be barely visible and can last from three to six months. Have a clear picture in your head and in your hand to show your stylist how you want to look so that your expectations are clear.

I slipped at a bus stop; I went one way and my hair went the other. That was the end of my wig.
~ Tia Carrere

Due to adhesives, hair extensions may not be appropriate for women with fine or fragile hair or for those that use scalp oils or relaxers. For African Americans, a good option for those who like the style is track braiding cornrows with human hair wefts. Hair extensions or weaves are also used in connection with hair transplant surgery.

Although expensive, getting the celebrity look is no longer just the domain of celebrities. Jessica Simpson and Raquel Welch have their own extension lines that you can check out at http://www.hairextensions.com. Doing research on the web to look for styles that might suit your face is a good way to start to define the look that you would like to achieve with extensions.

Hairpieces / Wigs

Hairpieces can be used to cover thinning or balding areas of the scalp and can be custom made. Hairpieces can be full or partial and may be composed of both natural and synthetic hair. Partial hair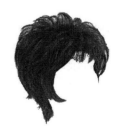

additions or nets are used for male- or female-pattern hair loss as well as for alopecia areata. Hairpieces are affixed to the scalp in several ways, including adhesive tapes and liquid adhesives. The scalp and hairpieces must be washed regularly and hairpieces loosen and fade over time, requiring replacement. Hairpieces can be a good option for women who are thinning as well as men with more prominent bald spots.

SURGICAL TREATMENTS

Hair Transplants

There are surgical techniques for replacing lost hair. Surgery may involve hair (skin and follicle) transplants or scalp reduction or some combination of both.

With hair transplants, areas of the scalp that have follicles producing hair are surgically removed and relocated to other parts of the scalp, such as the hairline or top of the head. Follicles or hair flaps are generally taken from the sides or back of the scalp. Transplants of one or two hairs are called "micrografts" but larger plugs of up to fifteen hairs may be used. Micrografts appear to have a higher success rate for transplantation. Follicles taken from areas of vigorously growing hair are more likely to yield a successful result. Use of synthetic hair fibers has been banned by the FDA due to the resulting high infection rate.

For a walk through the surgical process, consider reading *Patient's Guide to Hair Restoration*, a booklet written by surgeons who specialize in hair loss treatment and transplant surgery. The booklet

is available online free in PDF format at
http://www.newhair.com/resources/medical-publications.asp.

Hair transplant technology may eventually include more than hair follicles. A British firm, Intercytex has been experimenting since 2002 with transplanting dermal papilla cells. Dermal papilla cells are specialized tissue that reside at the base of the hair follicle and provide the follicle with glucose and amino acids for the production of hair.

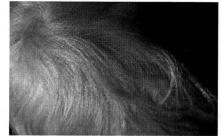

Naming their procedure "TrichoCyte," Intercytex scientists hope to formulate a procedure for widespread use that, like hair transplant surgery, removes dermal papilla from a less noticeable portion of the scalp, such as the side of the head. The scalp flap is then processed to isolate dermal papilla cells that are then injected into more prominent balding areas on the scalp. Research into this technology continues.

Scalp Reduction

Scalp reduction is surgically performed to decrease the appearance of a bald scalp. Scalp reduction is usually done in combination with either hair transplant or hair flap surgery. Alternatively, there are devices that can be used to stretch areas of the scalp where hair is still growing, increasing the appearance of a fuller head of hair. The success of these types of surgery depends on the amount of hair already lost and the elasticity of the skin on the scalp.

I'm a big woman. I need big hair.
~ Aretha Franklin

As noted, surgical methods are generally expensive and can be painful. Between 50 and 70 individual grafts may be needed to create a new hairline and the process is time consuming, sometimes up to two years. Scarring, surgical complications or infection may result and transplanted follicles may or may not continue to produce hair over time.

The importance of finding a qualified, experienced surgeon cannot be underestimated when considering hair transplant surgery. Check with your dermatologist for referrals. When you find a surgeon, ask for pictures of their work and for references to former clients who have used your surgeon in the past. Speaking with former patients can give you a good idea of what to expect as well as whether you've found the right surgeon.

DEALING WITH YOUR THYROID-RELATED HAIR LOSS

Many people notice rapid hair loss as a symptom of thyroid problems, and especially, hypothyroidism. Some people actually say this is the worst symptom of their thyroid problem -- this thinning hair, large amounts falling out in the shower or sink, often accompanied by changes in the hair's texture, making it dry, coarse, or easily tangled. Interestingly, some thyroid problems are even "diagnosed" at first by hairdressers, who notice the change in a client's hair!

It's important to understand that hair loss in linked to thyroid problems in five ways:

Thyroid problems can trigger Telogen Effluvium/TE

Having an overactive or underactive thyroid can trigger general shedding of hair throughout the head, and, in some cases, some loss of body hair (i.e., underarm and public hair.) You'll often notice more hair in drains and in the shower, in hair brushes, and when you brush your hair, but there are no specific patches of loss or even baldness.

A characteristic sign of an underactive thyroid, however, is loss of the hair from the outer edge of the eyebrow. TE is a common form of hair loss for people with undiagnosed or untreated thyroid disease.

Some thyroid hormone replacement drugs can trigger Telogen Effluvium/TE

While it seems odd, some *treatments* for an underactive thyroid – the thyroid hormone replacement drug levothyroxine in particular – can actually cause hair loss. They've taken it off their drug insert in recent years, but as of several years ago, Synthroid's patient insert had the following notice:

> **"Partial hair loss may occur during the initial months of therapy, but is generally transient. The incidence of continued hair loss is unknown."**

So while hair loss may have been a symptom of your underactive thyroid, the medication you take to treat the thyroid condition can continue or worsen the hair loss problem.

http://www.thyroid-info.com/hair

Be aware, however that many doctors do NOT know this, so don't be surprised if your doctor says that hair loss has nothing to do with your thyroid medication.

How you lose or keep your hair depends on how wisely you choose your parents.
~ Edward Nida

The autoimmune disease Alopecia Areata is more common on autoimmune thyroid patients

Even if you are diagnosed, and treated for Hashimoto's disease or Graves' disease, the underlying autoimmunity does not typically go away. And some people have more than one autoimmune disease at the same time. Even if you don't have the characterist round patches, or total hair loss of alopecia, you may have a milder, borderline alopecia that is causing increased hair loss, despite thyroid treatment.

The hormonal imbalances of thyroid disease appear to aggravate Androgenetic Alopecia in some people.

In Androgenetic Alopecia/AGA -- male and female pattern hair loss -- an enzyme starts to convert the hormone testosterone on the scalp to its less useful version, dihydrotestosterone (DHT), which then triggers hair loss. While the mechanism is unclear, it appears that some thyroid patients, who already often reproductive hormone imbalances, including imbalances in estrogen, progesterone and testosterone, are more suspectible to an earlier or more severe onset of AGA.

The age when thyroid disease often appears, in our late 40s and older, also coincides with increased rates of Androgenetic Alopecia

The risk of having a thyroid condition increases substantially at age 50 and beyond. At the same time, according to the American Academy of Dermatology, men have a 50 percent chance of experiencing AGA by age 50, and AGA is seen in up to 25 percent of pre-menopausal women and in 38 percent of post-menopausal women.

So, while the thyroid condition is not causing the AGA, "normal" AGA-related hair loss may be aggravated or worsened by a thyroid condition. And, thyroid-related hair loss that occurs at the same time as the AGA may make the overall hair loss more noticeable.

PRACTICAL STEPS

If Your Thyroid Problem Is Untreated, Get Diagnosed and Treated

If you're experiencing hair loss and are just starting treatment for a thyroid condition, it's likely that the loss will slow down, and eventually stop, once hormone levels are stabilized and your TSH levels fall within the new recommended normal range (0.3 to 3.0).

THYROID GUIDE TO HAIR LOSS

See a Dermatologist to Determine the Nature of Your Hair Loss

It's important to determine what type of hair loss you have. If you have alopecia areata, for example, that will determine the range of options available to you for treatment, vs. androgenic alopecia. A dermatologist can prescribe hair loss drugs (such as finasteride/Propecia), or recommend other medical treatments.

The dermatologist can also perform testing for nutritional deficiencies and hormonal imbalances that contribute to hair loss.

If Hair Loss Continues, Optimize Your TSH Level and Thyroid Drug

If you've gotten diagnosed and treated, and given yourself several months with your thyroid stabilized, and your hair loss continues, or worsens, then some of the things to consider:

- You may need to be at a different TSH level to minimize your symptoms
- You may be sensitive to your levothyroxine, and switching to the hypoallergenic 50 mcg. size pill of the levothyroxine medication could help
- You might respond better to the addition to T3 to your treatment
- You might respond better to a natural desiccated thyroid drug, i.e., Armour

http://www.thyroid-info.com/hair

Consider Supplementing With Evening Primrose Oil

When I have had major bouts of hair loss (despite optimized TSH and being on a T4/T3 drug), I took the advice of noted thyroid experts. In his book, *Solved: The Riddle of Illness*, Stephen Langer, M.D. points to the fact that symptoms of essential fatty acid insufficiency are very similar to hypothyroidism, and recommends evening primrose oil -- an excellent source of essential fatty acids -- as helpful for people with hypothyroidism. The usefulness of evening primrose oil, particularly in dealing with the issues of excess hair loss with hypothyroidism, was also reinforced by endocrinologist Kenneth Blanchard. According to Dr. Blanchard:

> For hair loss, I routinely recommend multiple vitamins, and especially evening primrose oil. If there's any sex pattern to it -- if a woman is losing hair in partly a male pattern - -then, the problem is there is excessive conversion of testosterone to dihydrotestosterone at the level of the hair follicle. Evening primrose oil is an inhibitor of that conversion. So almost anybody with hair loss probably will benefit from evening primrose oil.

I can vouch for the fact that taking evening primrose oil definitely helped caml down my hair loss at its worst.

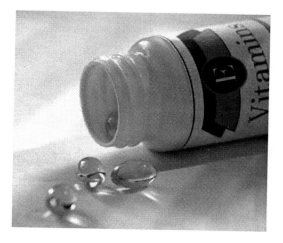

It slowed, then stopped the loss. The hair quality changed, and became less tangly and coarse. My hair was no longer straw-like.

Then the hair started to regrow, first

as very thin hairs mainly around the hairline, and later, regular hair.

It takes time though, so give yourself at least 4 to 5 months taking the EPO to start expecting signs that it's working.

When I take evening primrose oil, I usually take from 1000 to 2500 mg a day.

Consider Minoxidil (Rogaine)

During periods of shedding, minoxidil may be able to help prevent loss of some of the hair that you do have. You need to use it twice a day for least four months before results are typically seen. Minoxidil is available over the counter without a prescription.

Nutrition and Supplements

In terms of our diet, make sure you're getting enough protein and iron in your diet, as deficiencies in both can trigger hair loss.

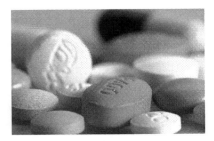

You should consider adding a good quality multivitamin that includes zinc. You may also want to add a good B-complex supplement.

Also consider supplemental saw palmetto, lysine and arginine, or a combination hair loss formula that includes these supplements.

Alternative Approaches

You may want to look for a practicioner to follow an alternative/integrative therapy such as Ayurveda, Chinese Medicine, acupuncture, aromatherapy

Typically, such a practitioner will not address just your hair loss, but your overall health, to help resolve the underlying issues.

Try a Self-Help Mind-body Approach

Learning techniques such as biofeedback and self-hypnosis can help, not only in stress reduction, but can have benefits for the immune system, and ma help with hair loss

An excellent and effective program for biofeedback and relaxation that you can use at home on your personal computer is Natural Rhythms from Wild Divine (http://www.wilddivine.com).

A highly-regarded expert on medical hypnotism is Dr. Steven Gurgevich. Any of his stress-relief audio sessions, which you can purchase online at http://www.tranceformation.com, may be helpful.

Consider Hair Care Products

Consider purchasing gentle shampoos, conditioners and volumizers at your local drugstore. While not affecting the amount of your hair, these inexpensive products can improve the texture and appearance of hair. Shampoos cleanse the scalp while conditioners coat the hair shaft to improve shine and deter breakage. Volumizers can be useful in hiding the effects of thinning. Sprayed toward the base of the hair shaft, volumizers give the appearance of thicker, fuller hair which, along with a good hair cut, can go a long way to disguising the thinner hair experienced as we age.

One product I particularly recommend is Pantene's Breakage Defense line, which is especially helpful when you're experiencing dry, breaking or tangling hair.

HAIR LOSS HOPE IN THE FUTURE

Research into hair loss continues, and there will no doubt be more drugs and treatments on the horizon.

Alopecia areata, is a promising area. A five-year study recently published in the *Journal of Investigative Dermatology* reports that researchers were able to identify a mouse with AA whose disease was almost identical to adult human AA. The study found that AA is, as suspected, a complicated condition involving four or more genes. Being able to reproduce the disease in a mouse model means that treatments and causative factors for AA can be studied in greater depth. Other research into AA, including the AA Gene Hunting Research Project, looks at gene mapping. These studies look at hair follicle development and biology, the development of new medications to treat autoimmune disorders and new ways of delivering those drugs.

New clinical trials are always in the works as well. For specific information about upcoming clinical trials, go to http://clinicaltrials.gov/ and search on the term "alopecia areata."

There is a silver lining in the fact that hair loss is a common malady for which people will pay for relief. The research and commercial hair loss industry is ever-reaching to find new solutions for hair loss problems, always searching for that "magic bullet."

To that end, the future couldn't be brighter. Despite the complexity of the mechanism of hair loss, science continues to search for the factors beyond dihydrotestosterone that cause male- and female-pattern hair loss.

Recent research published in the journal *Nature* has shed light on a theory first propounded fifty years ago that hair follicles regenerate after wounding. This almost forgotten theory, along with modern molecular science, led to the discovery that the loss of hair follicles, once thought to be permanent, may not be. By using mice that had been genetically altered to produce a higher level of a signaling protein, researchers found that the mice developed new hair follicles. The new follicles eventually produced hair identical to that located in nearby, unwounded areas.

Development of this research might lead to new techniques of treating hair loss, such as some sort of dermabrasion combined with a topical cream to reproduce the high signaling protein levels engineered in the mouse experiment. This finding and the research to follow will likely lead to a new understanding of alopecia and indeed, of the power and intricacy of the body's natural healing process.

Further insight into estrogens, signaling pathways and chemical communication might yield improved pharmaceutical products and treatments that may better arrest and reverse the hair loss process. Genetic research may offer up the secrets to the causation and better management of autoimmune disorders such as alopecia areata.

In the meantime, take heart, you are not alone. Hair loss has been around since there has been hair. Some of the treatments described in this guide may or may not be suitable for you, but we are living in a time when hair loss need not be an embarrassing secret. If you are concerned or depressed about hair loss, see a qualified doctor or dermatologist. Log onto the web, chances are you will find a discussion group, List or blog about the type of hair loss you may have. Talk to people, get information, but most of all – keep your head up. Like genetic patterns, you are unique and you have your own path to walk – with or without your hair.

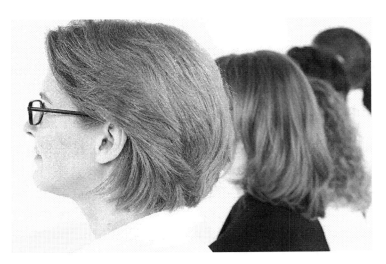

APPENDIX:
FINDING A HAIR LOSS EXPERT

SHOULD I SEE A DOCTOR?

To many, hair loss is a natural part of the aging process and despite the occasional anguished frustration in the mirror, or when viewing old photographs, the anxiety generally passes. There are signs though, that signal you should contact a qualified doctor or dermatologist right away.

If your hair suddenly begins to fall out in clumps or patches or if you experience redness, flaking or pain of the scalp, you should contact your doctor for an examination. As well, if you are a woman under 30 and your hair begins to shed and thin significantly (your ponytail becomes thin and you can see your scalp more easily when styling), you should make the call as well. Some women with high testosterone levels may experience abnormal menstrual periods, deepening of the voice and male-pattern hair growth (face and chest)

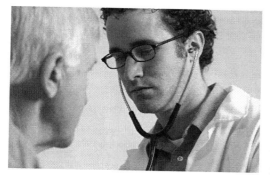

and thus male-pattern hair loss. If you have these symptoms, contacting your doctor for a check-up is warranted, if only to give you an idea of what to expect in the future.

For women and men, if you experience thinning and generalized shedding of your hair, this may be the

http://www.thyroid-info.com/hair

first sign of a thyroid disorder. Contact your doctor for an examination and be sure to mention your hair loss and any other symptoms you might be having. Correction of an underlying physical disorder may restore your hair, whereas waiting and wondering will cause only worry. The earlier that you notice and seek assistance with your concern over hair loss, the better chance you have of slowing or stopping some types of hair loss.

If the main symptoms you are having are depression or anxiety or hair loss – those are good reasons to contact your doctor as well. Your doctor or a qualified dermatologist can give you the information you need and provide referrals.

HOW DO YOU FIND A HAIR LOSS EXPERT?

A dermatologist is an expert in diagnosing and treating all types of hair loss. After initial examination by your own doctor, he or she may be able to provide you with a referral to a qualified dermatologist in your area who can treat the type of hair loss you may be experiencing.

The American Academy of Dermatologists is a professional organization that had its beginnings in the late 19th and early 20th centuries. It is the largest dermatologic association in the United States and offers a variety of public information on its website, located at http://www.aad.org. You can locate a dermatologist who is a member of the American Academy of Dermatologists by visiting the AAD website or by calling their toll free public information line at (888) 462-3376.

THYROID GUIDE TO HAIR LOSS

You can also contact your city, county or state medical societies for referrals to a qualified doctor or dermatologist.

Another type of expert you might consult with is called a "trichologist." A trichologist is a hair and scalp specialist, not a doctor. However, he or she can be qualified, much like a medical assistant, to carry out evaluations and make non-pharmacological recommendations. A directory of trichologists is maintained by the Trichological Society, at their website at http://www.hairscientists.org/regions.htm.

WHAT TYPES OF TESTS CAN YOU EXPECT DURING A HAIR LOSS EVALUATION?

As with all visits to a doctor's office, make sure that you write down and take in a list of questions and concerns that you may have. By writing questions down in advance, you can be sure that all your questions are addressed during your office visit.

During your visit to a doctor or specialist, you may expect to provide information on your medical and family history, your current physical condition, diet and nutritional habits, hair care habits and information on any medications (including vitamins and herbal supplements) you might be taking.

Along with a scalp examination, the doctor may ask you to monitor hairs lost during a day. She or he may collect a few hairs (called a "pull" test) and may perform a small scalp biopsy (a procedure performed in the doctor's office that is very useful for determining types of hair loss) for examination under a microscope and evaluation of hair condition, growing stage and hair shaft miniaturization.

As noted, be sure that you always insist on comprehensive thyroid bloodwork to rule out a thyroid condition as the cause of your thyroid disease.

Depending upon the doctor and what they observe, they may suggest blood tests for testosterone, estrogen, progesterone, parathyroid, iron, vitamin B-12 and calcium levels. Along with that they may suggest a complete blood count (CDC) blood screen. Additional tests may screen for syphilis (which causes hair loss as a secondary symptom) and ANA (for lupus which can cause generalized hair loss).

> **A visit to a qualified expert can set aside some of your worries, give you information you can use and possibly avoid the frustrating emotional consequences of continued hair loss.**

APPENDIX: RESOURCES

American Academy of Dermatology
PO Box 4014
Schaumburg, IL 60618-4014
Phone: (847) 330-0230 / Toll Free: (888) 462-3376 (Public Information System)
Fax: (847) 330-0050
http://www.aad.org
Find a Dermatologist search page:
http://www.aad.org/public/searchderm.htm
Find a Dermatologist Toll-free: 888-462-DERM

American Hair Loss Association
23679 Calabasas Road # 254
Calabasas, CA 91301-1502
http://www.americanhairloss.org

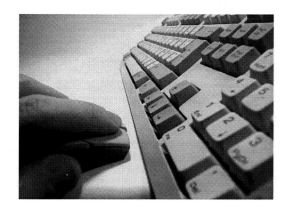

Spencer Kobren, The Bald Truth
Web site and radio show
http://thebaldtruth.com

American Society of Plastic Surgeons
444 E. Algonquin Road
Arlington Heights, IL 60005
Toll Free: (888) 475-2784
http://www.plasticsurgery.org

Hair Loss Scams
http://www.hairlossscams.com/index.html
A short, easy to read reference to hair loss scams

National Institute of Arthritis and Musculoskeletal and Skin Diseases
(NIAMS)
National Institutes of Health
1 AMS Circle
Bethesda, MD 20892-3675
(301) 495-4484 or 1-877-22-NIAMS (1-877-226-4267)
E-mail: NIAMSInfo@mail.nih.gov
http://www.niams.nih.gov

National Center for Complementary and Alternative Medicine
Clearinghouse
P.O. Box 7923
Gaithersburg, MD 20898
(301) 519-3153 or 1-888-644-6226
E-mail: info@nccam.nih.gov
http://nccam.nih.gov

National Alopecia Areata Foundation
14 Mitchell Boulevard
San Rafael, CA 94903
(415) 472-3780
Email: info@naaf.org
http://www.naaf.org

Cicatricial Alopecia Research Foundation
PO Box 64158
Los Angeles, CA 90064
Email: info@carfintl.org
http://www.carfintl.org/index.html

Hair Loss Talk.Com
http://www.hairlosstalk.com/
A consumer hair loss resource

About.com Hair Loss
http://hairloss.about.com
News/Information on Hair Loss

APPENDIX: REFERENCES

American Academy of Dermatology, www.aad.org

American Medical Association, http://www.ama-assn.org/

National Alopecia Areata Foundation, http://www.naaf.org

Mouse Model Gives Insight to Human Hair Loss, Journal of Investigative Dermatology November, Commentary, 2004

Hirsutism, Postpartum Telogen Effluvium, and Male Pattern Alopecia, Journal of Cosmetic Dermatology, 5, 81-86

Onion juice (Allium cepa L.), a new topical treatment for alopecia areata, Journal of Dermatology, 2002 Jun;29(6):343-6.

Advances in the Treatment of Male Androgenetic Alopecia: a Brief Review of Finasteride Studies, European Journal of Dermatology, 2001 Jul-August 11(4):332-4

Depression Circumstantially Related to the Administration of Finasteride for Androgenetic Alopecia, Journal of Dermatology, 2002 October; 29(10):665-9

THYROID GUIDE TO HAIR LOSS

Finasteride Treatment of Patterned Hair Loss in Normoandrogenic Postmenopausal Women, Dermatology, 2004, Vol. 209, No. 3

Skin Deep; At Hair Salons, an Extension on Youth, Elizabeth Hayt, The New York Times, September 28, 2006

Burden of Hair Loss: Stress and the Underestimated Psychosocial Impact of Telogen Effluvium and Androgenetic Alopecia, Journal of Investigative Dermatology, 123: 455-457, 2004

Randomized Trial of Aromatherapy – Successful Treatment for Alopecia Areata, Archives of Dermatology, 1998, 134:1349-1352

The Hair Follicle as an Estrogen Target and Source, Endocrine Review, 2006 Oct; 27(6):677-706

In Search of the "Hair Cycle Clock": a Guided Tour, Differentiation, 72:489-511

A Randomized, Double-Blind, Placebo-Controlled Trial to Determine the Effectiveness of Botanically Derived Inhibitors of 5AR in the Treatment of Androgenetic Alopecia, Journal of Alternative and Complementary Medicine, Volume 8, Number 2, April 2002

Alopecia: Unapproved Treatments or Indications, Clinics in Dermatology, Volume 18, Issue 2, Pages 177-186

Journal of Investigative Dermatology Symposium Proceedings (2003) 8, 18–19; doi:10.1046/j.1523-1747.2003.12166.x

THYROID GUIDE TO HAIR LOSS

Wnt-dependent de novo hair follicle regeneration in adult mouse skin after wounding, Nature, Volume 447/17 May 2007/doi:10.1038/nature 05766

Nutritional factors and hair loss, Clinical and Experimental Dermatology 2002 Jul; 27(5):396-404

The diagnosis and treatment of iron deficiency and its potential relationship to hair loss, Journal of the American Academy of Dermatology. 2006 May; 54(5):824-44

Green Tea and Hair Loss, HairlossTalk.com, May 26, 2004, editorial by Dr. M. Sawaya (last accessed May, 2007)

Biofeedback, cognitive-behavioral methods, and hypnosis in dermatology: is it all in your mind?, Dermatologic Therapy 2003;16(2):114-22

Hypnosis in Dermatology, Archives of Dermatology, 2000; 136:393-39
Hypnotherapeutic management of alopecia areata. Journal of the American Academy of Dermatology, Volume 55, Issue 2, Pages 233-237 R

Treatment of Alopecia with Chinese Herbs, Subhuti Dharmananda, Ph.D., Director, Institute for Traditional Medicine, Portland, Oregon, http://www.itmonline.org/arts/alopecia.htm (last accessed June, 2007)

Randomized trial of aromatherapy. Successful treatment for alopecia areata. Arch Dermatol. 134.11 (1998): 1349-1352.

THYROID GUIDE TO HAIR LOSS

Onion juice (Allium cepa L.), a new topical treatment for alopecia areata. J Dermatol. 29.6 (2002): 343-346.

Hypnotherapeutic management of alopecia areata. J Am Acad Dermatol. 55.2 (2006): 233-237.

The PUVA-turban as a new option of applying a dilute psoralen solution selectively to the scalp of patients with alopecia areata. J Am Acad Dermatol. 2001 Feb;44(2):248-52.

The application of antioxidants in investigations and optimization of photochemotherapy. Membr Cell Biol. 1998;12(2):269-78.

APPENDIX:
MORE THYROID HELP

Once you're hypothyroid, you're hypothyroid for life. Because doctors simply don't have the time to stay up on all the latest developments, this is something you need to do, for you own well-being, quality of life, and health.

Free Email Newsletters

So you need reliable, easy ways to stay informed about thyroid disease. That's why you'll want to sign up for my FREE email newsletters.

Sticking Out Our Necks: The Thyroid Disease News Report, is a free monthly email newsletter that provides quick recaps of all the latest thyroid news, and links to important news stories on the web.

Sign up for email newsletters by going to
http://www.thyroid-info.com/newsletters.htm.

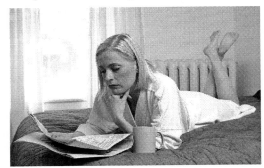

A Weight Off My Mind: Thyroid Diet & Weight Loss News Report, is a free monthly email newsletter that provides information on weight loss, metabolism, nutrition, and diet, all with an eye toward thyroid patients who are trying to eat healthy, lose weight, and stay slim.

Sticking Out Our Necks: Print Edition by Mail

The email newsletters are a great, quick resource. But many people want something more – they want in-depth coverage of the latest thyroid news, interviews and articles, information about little-known drug recalls, and the latest research released, along with many other features that have an impact on your thyroid condition, and your weight loss efforts.

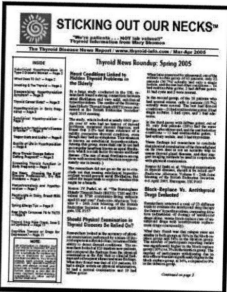

If that sounds like you, then you'll want to subscribe to the mail edition of *Sticking Out Our Necks.* This print newsletter, which is published every other month, and delivered to your mailbox, is the only newsletter dedicated to your condition -- thyroid disease.

If you subscribe, you'll never have to worry about whether key health research on thyroid disease has come out and you've missed it. You'll know that every other month, you're going to get 12 pages of the latest findings about thyroid disease, delivered to your mailbox, and all you have to do it sit back and read.

Here are some subscribers' thoughts about the newsletter:

THYROID GUIDE TO HAIR LOSS

For the first time since my diagnosis in 1999, I feel like my old self again. Mary, if it wasn't for you, I would still be settling for a life of under treated Hashimoto's disease. Instead, I am enjoying high levels of energy and desire. For the first time in years, I am experiencing hopes, dreams, and a vision for what I can accomplish in life. And, just as important, I have the physical, emotional, and mental energy to reinvent my life. What joy I experience when some of my friends and family don't recognize the new me!

~ Heidi H, Asheville, NC

You have given me the confidence to fight for feeling well, a valuable service to anyone, and, surely, a human right. I am now slim, my TSH is rock bottom of range and I have never had as many compliments from people - I look and feel 10 years younger than I did 18 months ago. I know I'm one of the lucky ones, but it isn't ALL luck: I've followed your advice and it's paid off.

~Alison L, London, England

What you are doing is commendable. Someone helping others, even while in the midst of their own struggle is a rare gift seldom found in people. I'm sure there are many who appreciate all that you do. Thank you, and I hope your message continues to reach and empower others.

~ Don G.

You did a great job and thank you for all the hard work you put into it. There is so much information that you gave this reader and follower more than her money's worth.

~ Lauren Y, Milwaukee, WI

A second opinion consultation with a doctor can cost $150 for a 15 minute visit. Just one hardcover book on health can cost you $24.95.

Yet, your total subscription cost for one year is only $25! ($35 non-US)

And this newsletter could easily sell for much more. Many specialized health newsletters cost as much as $179 a year!

But a year's worth of my newsletter -- that's 72 pages (and usually more, with special free extra inserts -- filled with news, information and specific help for thyroid patients is only $25 a year.

I currently charge $100 an hour just for a phone consultation. So at the bare minimum, since I spend weeks researching and writing each issue, you're getting hundreds of dollars worth of thyroid information and advice in each issue.)

$25 is a tiny investment, when compared to the health improvement potential you'll find in each issue.

If you are truly serious about living well despite your thyroid disease...then you won't want to overlook this opportunity to sign up, and start getting information that helps you get well and live well.

Your cost is peanuts compared to all the money you're probably going to save by not buying health newsletters and magazines that don't cover the health issues you face day to day. So that means...

You really can't afford not to sign up today!

Don't put this off. While all of this is fresh in your mind, do yourself a favor and order. It's easy!

ONLINE: go to **http://www.thyroid=info.com/subscribe.htm** to order quickly and securely online, using any major credit card.

FAX: Fill out the Order Form, and fax it, anytime, 24 hours a day, to 425-977-1175

MAIL: Pop your completed order form in the mail to me:
Mary Shomon, Thyroid-Info
PO Box 565
Kensington, MD 20895-0565

TOLL-FREE PHONE: Or give a toll-free call to the office at 1-888-810-9471 to order by phone, with any major credit card. (Make sure you mention your 2 free bonus issues!!)

Before you put this aside, take action now -- chances are too great you'll forget about all the immense health potential this newsletter can bring you.

Do You Find Yourself Saying: "I Wish I Knew Who to Call to Help Answer My Thyroid Questions...NOW!?"

If you're worried about your health...about finding the right doctor...difficulty getting diagnosed...thyroid symptoms that aren't going away...where to find answers to hard questions about thyroid disease and your health, I have an option you should seriously consider.

Let's face it, most doctors don't have the time to brainstorm with us about what conventional and treatment approaches ideas to research, or where to go for the best thyroid treatment. How can you get the information you deserve?

I can help.

In a one-on-one telephone coaching consultation, we'll brainstorm your thyroid questions, and I'll share ideas and resources with you on where to get more help so you can feel and live well.

If you have just one or two questions, then we can have a 15-minute consultation. If you have a whole list of things to discuss, sessions are available in 15 minute increments, up to an hour. Just the two of us, on the phone, brainstorming practical -- maybe even life-changing -- solutions to your health challenges.

You are invited to set up a phone consultation -- usually, I can schedule your session within a week -- to explore your thyroid questions, and map out a plan to help you enjoy better health. You have important questions, and getting answers is a key step that can help you tackle your thyroid problems and improve your health.

One important reminder -- since I'm NOT a doctor, I cannot offer specific medical advice. But I can and will guide you to resources, experts, information sources and more that will help you feel better!

You can book online now at **http://www.thyroidbreakthrough.com/contact.htm** or call toll-free 1-888-810-9471 to make your appointment with me now.

I look forward to speaking with you soon!

About Mary Shomon

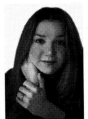 Mary Shomon is the nation's leading patient advocate on thyroid disease and the best-selling author of numerous books on thyroid, autoimmune and hormonal conditions. She is author of the New York Times bestselling book *The Thyroid Diet: Manage Your Metabolism for Lasting Weight Loss*" (2004) *Thyroid Diet* was also a semi-finalist for the prestigious Quills Awards in 2005, and an Amazon.com Top Ten Health Book of the Year.

Her best-selling, internationally-published book *Living Well with Hypothyroidism: What Your Doctor Doesn't Tell You...That You Need to Know*, was first published in 2000, and after more than 20 printings, a second edition came out in 2005. The book was a Prevention Book Club Selection, and Amazon.com Top-Selling health book, and its popularity launched a new series of consumer health books for publisher HarperCollins.

Mary Shomon is also author of *Thyroid Hormone Breakthrough* (2006), *Living Well With Graves' Disease and Hyperthyroidism*, (2005), *Living Well With Autoimmune Disease*,(2003) *Living Well With Chronic Fatigue Syndrome and Fibromyalgia*, (2004). Information about all of Mary Shomon's books and information resources is online at http://www.thyroid-info.com/bookstore.htm

Mary's newsletter for thyroid patients, *Sticking Out Our Necks,* was founded in 1997, and has become a popular resource for patients in both its email and print form.. Mary Shomon has served as the Guide for the popular About.com Thyroid site -- now part of the New York Times Company -- launching the site in early 1997, and managing the site and working as its sole researcher/writer since that time. That site, http://thyroid.about.com along with her advocacy site http://www.thyroid-info.com
are the Internet's most popular and visited sites dedicated to thyroid disease.

Mary Shomon has been featured in hundreds of television, radio, newspaper, magazine and web interviews, including appearances on ABC World News Tonight and CBS Radio Networks, and interviews in the *New York Times, Wall Street Journal, Ladies Home Journal, Health, Cooking Light, Elle Magazine, Woman's World*, and the *Los Angeles Times*, to name just a few.

In her decade of consumer advocacy, Mary Shomon has never hesitated to take a stand on behalf of patients, and her independence from drug companies and medical/patient organizations that are funded by the pharmaceutical industry has allowed her to maintain an unbiased, truly patient-first advocacy effort that is rare in the thyroid community.

Mary Shomon – On the Web

Mary Shomon can be found on the web at:
- Thyroid-Info.com – The Thyroid Disease Information Source http://www.thyroid-info.com

- Thyroid Site at About.com, a *New York Times* Company
  http://thyroid.about.com
- *Sticking Out Our Necks: Thyroid Disease News Report* – Email Newsletter
- *Weight Off My Mind: Thyroid & Autoimmune Disease Weight Loss/Metabolism News* – Email Newslette
  http://www.thyroidbreakthrough.com/newsletters.htm

Books by Mary J. Shomon
http://www.thyroidbreakthrough.com/bookstore.htm

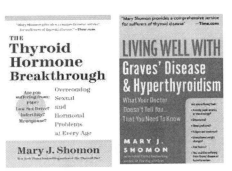 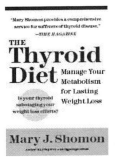 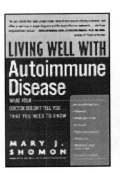 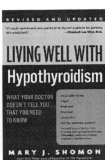

The Thyroid Hormone Breakthrough, Overcoming Sexual and Hormonal Problems at Every Age, 2006, HarperCollins

Living Well With Hypothyroidism: What Your Doctor Doesn't Tell You That You Need to Know, 2nd edition 2005, HarperCollins

---

http://www.thyroid-info.com/hair

Living Well With Graves' Disease and Hyperthyroidism: What Your Doctor Doesn't Tell You That You Need to Know, 2005, HarperCollins
The Thyroid Diet: Manage Your Metabolism for Lasting Weight Loss, 2004, HarperCollins

Living Well With Chronic Fatigue Syndrome and Fibromyalgia: What Your Doctor Doesn't Tell You That You Need to Know, 2004, HarperCollins

Living Well With Autoimmune Disease: What Your Doctor Doesn't Tell You That You Need to Know, 2002, HarperCollins

Living Well With Hypothyroidism: What Your Doctor Doesn't Tell You That You Need to Know, 1st edition 2000, HarperCollins

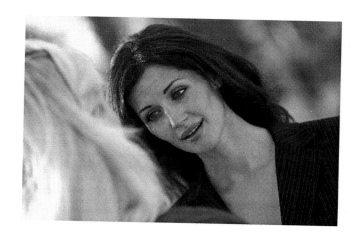

http://www.thyroid-info.com/hair

ORDER THE PRINT NEWSLETTER

☑ YES...I Want to Stay Informed About The Latest Thyroid News and Developments

_____ Sticking Out Our Necks Newsletter, 1-Year Subscription, US (6 bi-monthly 12-pg issues), $25

_____ Sticking Out Our Necks Newsletter, One-Year Subscription, Non-US Delivery*, $35*

*No checks in foreign currency for non-US orders please, credit cards or money orders in US dollars only

_____ Credit Card   or   _____ Check (Make check payable to "Sticking Out Our Necks")

Name:	Email:
Address:	Phone: (req'd if you're using a credit card)
City	State
Country	Zip/Postal Code

Credit Card Information: _____ VISA _____ MasterCard _____ American Express _____ Discover	Expiration Date:
Card Number:	Signature:

http://www.thyroid-info.com/hair

MAIL order form to:

Sticking Out Our Necks Newsletter Order
PO Box 565
Kensington, MD 20895-0565

FAX order form to…

425-977-1175

Phone…

Toll free 1-888-810-9471

Online…

http://www.thyroid-info.com/subscribe.htm

Please allow at least 3-4 weeks for delivery in the U.S.

Please note: We value your privacy, and do not sell your information or make it available to anyone.

NOTES